# MEMORY BOOKS

## *and Other Graphic Cuing Systems*

PRACTICAL COMMUNICATION AND MEMORY AIDS FOR ADULTS WITH DEMENTIA

**Michelle S. Bourgeois,** PH.D., CCC-SLP

Department of Communication Disorders
The Florida State University
Tallahassee, Florida

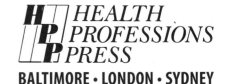

HEALTH
PROFESSIONS
PRESS

**BALTIMORE · LONDON · SYDNEY**

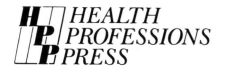

HEALTH
PROFESSIONS
PRESS

Health Professions Press, Inc.
Post Office Box 10624
Baltimore, Maryland 21285-0624

www.healthpropress.com

Designed and Produced by Columbia Publishing Services, Columbia, Maryland.
Typeset by Circle Graphics, Columbia, Maryland.
Manufactured in the United States of America by
Versa Press, Inc., East Peoria, Illinois.

Some of the artwork appearing in this text is from the public access clip art files of Microsoft Office® and Yahoo®.

Artwork appearing on pages 23–24 reprinted by permission of Taylor & Francis Ltd, http://www.tandf.co.uk/journals. (From Bourgeois, M.S., Dijkstra, K., Burgio, L., & Allen-Burge, R. [2001]. Memory aids as an augmentative and alternative communication strategy for nursing home residents with dementia. *Augmentative and Alternative Communication, 17,* 196–209.)

Artwork appearing on pages 29 (Marian Manor), 41 (It Hurts on…), 42 (Feeling sad and sick), 48, 62, 67 (Going to the Bathroom), 68 (To Shave), 75, and 76 reprinted by permission of Attainment Company, Inc. (Verona, WI).

Artwork appearing on page 67 (Transfer from wheelchair to bed) reprinted by permission of Harcourt Assessment, Inc. (for Therapy Skill Builders), San Antonio, TX.

Library of Congress Cataloging-in-Publication Data

Bourgeois, Michelle S.
   Memory books and other graphic cuing systems : practical communication and memory aids
for adults with dementia / by Michelle S. Bourgeois.
      p. ; cm.
   Includes bibliographical references.
   ISBN 978-1-932529-22-7
   1. Dementia. 2. Dementia—Treatment. 3. Memory disorders. 4. Graphic arts—
Therapeutic use. I. Title.
   [DNLM: 1. Dementia. 2. Communication. 3. Cues. WM 220 B772m 2007]
   RC394.M46B68 2007
   616.8'3—dc22
                                           2007003990

# Contents

# Preface

Since the publication of *Enhancing the Conversations of Memory-Impaired Persons: A Memory Aid Workbook* in 1992, I have had the opportunity to conduct a series of studies investigating the usefulness of memory books with persons with dementia at different levels of severity. I have also explored variations of memory books, including different sizes and formats and different categories and topics of information. I have learned much from each individual with dementia, family member, professional, and lay caregiver who participated in the research studies over these years. To all of you—thank you! Your generosity and willingness to assist with these projects made the difference; together we discovered the best types of memory aids to use with specific individuals. We found out which problems could be addressed effectively by making a memory book page, reminder card, or memo board message. We created a variety of wearable and portable memory aids. We developed and tested several different training programs and types of training materials. This revised workbook is the culmination of many years of dedicated work by many individuals whose involvement in the projects was driven by personal hopes for their own family member or client with dementia and by their recognition of the needs of all people challenged by the memory loss associated with dementia.

None of this would have been possible without the support of the agencies that funded this research—the Alzheimer's Association and the National Institute on Aging—and the many colleagues who helped to conceptualize the research designs and methods, implement the procedures and collect the data, analyze and present the results at many national and international conferences, and write the publications for journals and book chapters. This community of scholars is unsurpassed in their dedication to the discovery of effective interventions for improving the quality of the lives of our clients with dementia, their families, and caregivers. It has been an honor to work with each and every one of you.

# Memory Aids for a Variety of Purposes: Beyond Conversation

Ours is a busy, fast-paced world full of names, faces, places, facts, and figures to remember and use. We have appointments to keep, phone numbers to call, important facts to remember—so many that we often experience memory overload. How many of us can function without our memory aids—calendars, appointment books, shopping lists, Post-it notes, small scraps of paper in a coat pocket or at the bottom of a purse? Many manufacturers are taking advantage of our inadequate memories by offering us technological substitutes, such as computers, calculators, personal digital assistants, and cell phones. In this age of computers, we depend on technology to augment our memory capacity.

If the average person is overworking his or her memory just to get through the day, imagine the challenges facing individuals for whom memory loss is one symptom of a larger problem. The purpose of this book is to describe the use of a memory strategy—the use of written cues—that has evolved as it has been researched with a variety of individuals and in various formats from memory wallets, memory books, and memory boards to reminder cards. The original motivation for the development of memory wallets and memory books was to enhance conversation. Persons with dementia reported having difficulty remembering words, the names of familiar persons and places, and the topic of a conversation. Their family added observations of withdrawal and depression, frustration and anger, and avoidance of conversational interactions in group situations. The apparent solution was to provide a collection of pictures and sentences that the person could read and that would remind him or her of specific people, places, and events to discuss. As reported in Bourgeois (1990, 1992b), individuals with mild to moderate dementia demonstrated immediate changes in the content of their conversations when reading aloud the memory wallet or book pages and elaborating on the topic. These improved conversations continued over time and in some cases for up to 24 and 30 months, despite continued cognitive decline. Serendipitously, caregivers reported the usefulness of a memory book page to resolve difficult behaviors such as repetitive questioning. This led to providing written answers to questions in a variety of places, from the memo board on the refrigerator to an index card carried in a purse to a self-adhesive note on the car dashboard.

As the idea of using written text to cue memory has spread, professionals have adopted this strategy for the functional goals addressed in therapy with their clients with memory loss. Goals related to orientation; communication of wants, needs, and safety; increasing activity and engagement in activities; and reducing challenging behaviors have been addressed successfully with a variety of written cues. Speech-language pathologists are spreading the word among their colleagues in physical therapy, occupational therapy, and nursing. Nursing assistants, in particular, have been the focus of specific training programs designed to provide them with a tool to make their interactions with the resident with dementia more satisfying and successful. As this strategy continues to be used and adapted to solve a variety of problems, the technology will evolve. In the meantime, this text is designed to provide the most current information about how to make and use written cues for a range of memory-related problems.

*Note: The artwork in this book comes from a variety of sources, including the author, Attainment Company (Verona, WI), and clip art available from Microsoft® and Yahoo®. Information about these and other sources for pictures appears in Appendix D.*

# CHAPTER 1

# Research Update: The Evolution of Memory Books

Memory loss is one symptom of many and various neurological disorders, from specific focal injury resulting in aphasia, to more pervasive damage from a traumatic head injury or dementia. Memory loss can be exhibited in a variety of ways, such as losing things around the house; failing to recognize familiar places or getting lost on a walk; rambling conversation about unimportant or irrelevant things; difficulty learning new skills such as a game; word retrieval problems; forgetting or confusing recent events, a story, or detailed instructions; and repeating the same question because you forgot the answer or that you already asked it.

A popular theory to explain the structure and organization of memory in the brain speculates that memory is organized into encoding, storage, and retrieval processes (Baddeley, 1995). Information to be remembered has to first enter the system through the senses (visual, auditory, tactile), then is held temporarily in a working memory or short-term memory place. In this holding area, the information is examined and comprehended; the auditory parts of the information are thought to be processed by an articulatory or phonological "loop" and the visual information is processed by a visuospatial "scratch pad" (Baddeley, 1992). At this point the person has to make a decision: either respond to the information or store it for later retrieval. Long-term storage is thought to contain declarative or explicit memories (such as semantic, episodic, and autobiographical facts) and nondeclarative or implicit memories (such as skills and habits acquired with practice over the lifetime). The complex interaction of encoding, storing, and retrieving information is thought to be controlled by a central executive system that seems to be particularly vulnerable to encoding and retrieval difficulties associated with neurological conditions such as dementia (Baddeley, 1992). The types of information that present the greatest challenges in dementia are those that require conscious encoding, or new learning. Episodic memories, such as what you ate for lunch, or the answer to the question you just asked, need to be recognized as important to store for later retrieval; overlearned or habitual memories, such as walking, playing the piano, or counting to 100, are more resistant to the effects of neurological disease because they have been stored and retrieved repeatedly over a lifetime, often unconsciously and without effort. Retrieval of memories from remote long-term storage is also relatively preserved; caregivers remark that persons may remember details from their childhood, but not the names of their own children. The challenge to families and rehabilitation professionals is to recognize and understand the type of memory problem presenting itself, and then find a way to remediate it.

In general, the research literature falls into three general approaches to the remediation of memory deficits. The first approach is to attempt to restore memory through repetitive drill and practice (Sohlberg & Mateer, 2001). It is assumed that with repetitive drill and practice the brain will compensate; intact areas will take over the functions and processes previously dedicated to the impaired area. Computer programs for retraining memory are based on the drill approach, but there is little evidence that gains in basic skills—such as attention, concentration, visual perception, simple memory, and organization—generalize to functional daily-life activities (Lynch, 2002; Sohlberg & Mateer, 2001). The current popularity of the "use it or lose it" theory by the general public is motivating people to do crossword puzzles, learn a new language, or memorize license plate numbers in order to prevent memory loss and dementia; the published research in this area is equivocal, however (Hultsch, Hertzog, Small, & Dixon, 1999; Mackinnon, Christensen, Hofer, Korten, & Jorm, 2003).

The second approach to remedy memory disorders is to teach the person to use a strategy for remembering desired information. Some of the more common strategies include visual imagery (picture-name and face-name associations, mental retracing of events, motor coding), mnemonics (rhyming peg, phonetic system, loci method), and verbal elaboration strategies (story linking, alphabetical cueing/chunking, first letter mnemonic, and lyrical strategies) (e.g., Fogler & Stern, 1988). These strategies provide an organizational structure for the information to be recalled and specific devices (or "tricks") to use to access the information. This approach assumes the person will learn a strategy that will improve memory functioning and, once trained, will use the strategy for a reasonable length of time. Unfortunately, there is scant evidence that many of these strategies are effective in the long run. In fact, the use of a strategy can place heavy demands on the already disordered cognitive system and may not be a realistic approach for all persons with memory impairment.

The third approach to remedy memory deficits is to provide a compensatory system, or memory prosthesis, in the form of a memory aid or cues. Some compensatory systems *substitute for* a memory function, such as an alarm clock, watch, or calendar; others *perform* a memory function, such as computer software and autodialing telephones. These types of compensatory systems relieve the additional burdens of knowing *how* to do something, *when* to do it, and, in some cases, the *additional details* (such as a telephone number) required to accomplish the task. A prosthetic environment is one in which stimuli and cues evoke and reinforce appropriate functional behavior, such as labels on cupboards and signs on the bathroom door. A wide variety of compensatory memory aids have been successful, including memory notebooks, bell timers and alarm clocks, written notes, shopping lists, tape-recorded messages, electronic organizers, a string on the finger, putting items in special places, and asking others to remind you (Bourgeois, 2006; Kapur, 1995). Practical suggestions abound, including: simplifying the environment, establishing a consistent daily routine of activities, providing "extra" stimuli (signs, labels, color codes, etc.), and practicing basic skills (reading labels, writing a signature, etc.). Researchers and clinicians have been conducting studies on a variety of these memory aids and the evidence for their effectiveness is appearing in the literature (Bourgeois, 2006); more research is still warranted, however.

The first experimentally validated memory aids developed for enhancing the conversations of persons with dementia were the **memory aid wallet** and **memory aid book** approaches (Bourgeois, 1990, 1992a, 1992b). Designed to present factual information in a written and picture format, memory aid wallets/books contained approximately 30 pages of information consisting of a single declarative sentence and a picture to illustrate the stated fact. The results of these studies documented the effectiveness of using written and picture cues to improve conversations of people with dementia. Bourgeois (1990) demonstrated that three women with middle-

stage Alzheimer's disease used a communication wallet to remind themselves of specific factual information when conversing with familiar conversational partners. Subjects participated in twice-daily sessions with their husbands during which they read aloud the sentences in their memory wallet. They not only increased the number of on-topic statements of fact made during 5-minute conversations, but they also decreased the number of ambiguous, erroneous, and perseverative utterances said during the same conversations with the experimenter and a familiar conversational partner (a neighbor or daughter). They maintained improved conversational performance at 3- and 6-week follow-up sessions after treatment termination. In a series of studies, memory aids were shown to enhance the conversations of persons with varying degrees of cognitive impairment (Bourgeois, 1991, 1992b), to support their pragmatic skills of turn-taking and topic initiation (Bourgeois, 1993), and to facilitate meaningful interactions among adult day service participants, staff, and volunteers (Bourgeois & Mason, 1996).

Specific characteristics of memory aids and implementation details were also a research focus. For example, the importance of the reading practice sessions was

investigated in Bourgeois (1992b); in Experiment 1, practice sessions were decreased from twice daily to once a day and similar effects on conversations were observed. When practice sessions were eliminated altogether in Experiment 2 and the effects of the memory aid were still evident on the conversations, Bourgeois proposed that training may not be needed for the desired reading behaviors. In fact, these reading skills may represent preserved skills in comparison to others that were documented to be declining during the same time period (e.g., MMSE scores). A study with persons with more severe manifestations of dementia symptoms appeared to support this claim. Bourgeois (1991) recruited eight subjects with cognitive deficits in the severe range from a long-term care nursing facility and provided them with memory aids in the $8\frac{1}{2} \times 11$–inch book format and enlarged print font. Treatment effects were mostly similar to results in prior studies; however, some of the lowest functioning subjects required some prompts to read the written statements and the degree to which they elaborated on the written statements varied by person.

These studies also documented the importance of constructing a memory aid whose physical characteristics—including size and type of pages, and size of the print font—matched the needs of the person with dementia who may have been experiencing sensory decline. Bourgeois (1992a) developed a five-item oral reading screening tool in two formats, a memory book (8½ × 11–inch page + 36-point font) and a wallet (3 × 5 inch + 14-point font). Each page had one simple declarative sentence and one line drawing to illustrate the sentence; the five sentences consisted of 24 words. This screening tool was used to evaluate oral reading performance with those particular memory aid formats and font sizes. The total number of words read correctly out of the 24 total possible was calculated; a score of <20 out of 24 indicated a larger font size was required. Observations of memory aid use and number and type of prompts required to encourage manipulation of the memory aid were helpful in prescribing the appropriate characteristics of the memory aid to be developed for a particular person.

An important observation was made by the husband of a subject who did not demonstrate measurable treatment effects; he noticed that his wife changed the tone of her vocalizations when looking at the memory book, smiled, and patted the pictures—behaviors that indicated to him that she recognized the people in the pictures and that this was pleasurable to her. This raises a measurement issue; the behaviors affected by familiar picture and written stimuli may include those not typically measured by speech-language pathologists (SLPs). In this example, this woman's vocalizations changed in affect, from agitated sounds to pleasant sounds; they were not identifiable words and certainly not the written statements in her book. The husband was adamant that the memory book was the most important therapeutic intervention she had received in recent weeks and one that he could use to improve the quality of her life. We may need to consider a wider range of outcome measures when attempting to document intervention effects with individuals with more severe impairment. Documenting changes in affect as a result of treatment may be an important focus of future research.

Other anecdotal reports of changes in difficult behaviors following memory book intervention have led to studies of the effects of written cues to document these changes. One husband in the Bourgeois (1990) study reported that the page in the memory wallet that illustrated the sentence, "I have lived in this house at 123 Elm Street for 54 years," was effective in reminding his wife that she was at home, thereby reducing her attempts to leave the house in the early evening (sun-downing behavior). Another caregiver requested a specific way to reduce her father's repeated requests for information about the return of his deceased wife; a page documenting the fact that his wife had died on a specific date with a picture of her gravesite was reported to reduce those questions. These observations led to the Bourgeois, Burgio, Schulz, Beach, and Palmer (1997) study in which the repeated verbalizations of home-dwelling persons with dementia were reduced by teaching the caregiver to provide a written response in the form of a memory book page, an index card, or a memo board. In each of seven cases, the written cue was effective at reducing the frequency of the repeated questions.

Once SLPs around the United States began to make memory books and wallets for their patients with dementia, reports of problems and frustrations surrounding the use of memory books in long-term care facilities began to surface. SLPs complained that the certified nursing assistants (CNAs) were reluctant to use the memory books they had developed for the resident in spite of in-service training efforts. It was common to visit a nursing home resident and notice a memory book lying unused in his or her room. Upon reflection of these complaints, two problems emerged. First, the memory books constructed by SLPs for their patients were often beautifully detailed albums consisting of 30 or more pages that resembled the type of photo album one would find on a coffee table in one's home. It seemed that SLPs were expecting CNAs and other nursing home personnel to take the time to have conversational interactions with residents using these memory books. When CNAs were interviewed about their perceptions of the memory books, they admitted it was a nice idea to have pictures and text describing the residents, their lives, and their families, but that they did not have the time to spend in such conversations. When CNAs were in resident rooms, they reported feeling constrained to focus their attention solely on the personal care activities they were required to accomplish with the resident, such as toileting, bathing, dressing, and grooming tasks. They did not know how to organize their schedules to have time for a personal conversation or to reminisce about the resident's past life. They mentioned that these memory books would be useful to residents during conversations with other residents, but that the books were too large for residents to easily transport by themselves to common room locations.

Two solutions surfaced. First, memory books needed to be smaller, lighter in weight, and easier for the resident to transport; they had the potential to be used to elicit conversations between residents in locations other than the resident's room if they could accompany the resident. Second, CNAs were not using memory books because they did not know how to incorporate them into their activities with the residents. Therefore, if the memory books contained pages that were pertinent to personal care activities and could be viewed as a means of making the task easier or quicker to accomplish, then they might be viewed as useful tools by the care staff.

Memory wallets were, therefore, modified to be lighter in weight by reducing the number of pages (from 30 to 12) and to include pages that addressed personal care activities for which the CNA was responsible and with which residents might be reluctant to cooperate. In addition, the idea that residents might want to use their memory aid in a location other than their room was addressed by devising ways for the memory aid to be attached to the resident or his or her walker/wheelchair. Appendix A provides patterns and instructions for making the types of devices that facilitated memory book availability wherever the resident might go, including necklaces, belts, wristbands, pocketed vests and aprons,

and walker/wheelchair bags. Bourgeois and colleagues were funded by the National Institute on Aging ("Increasing Effective Communication in Nursing Homes," AG 13008-01, 1996–2000) to evaluate a training program for CNAs that involved teaching them to use memory aids during personal care activities in order to enhance communication with residents with dementia. In this randomized, treatment versus control group designed study, CNAs who received training in the use of memory aids and other communication skills with their residents with dementia talked more, used more positive statements, and used more specific instructions with residents in comparison with CNAs who did not receive this training. The residents with memory aids had more positive verbal interactions with staff, visitors, and other residents as a result of the intervention (Allen-Burge, Burgio, Bourgeois, Sims, & Nunnikhoven, 2001; Burgio et al., 2001; Bourgeois, Dijkstra, Burgio, & Allen-Burge, 2001). Nursing assistants reported satisfaction with using the memory aid during personal care activities, stating they could use it either to help the resident understand what care activity was about to occur, or to help distract the resident during the activity by discussing some personal information depicted in the memory aid.

The success of this study led to the development of additional training materials for direct-care staff in the form of an interactive CD-ROM computer software package comprised of four modules, one specifically designed to teach the use of written cues during personal care activities. Bourgeois and Irvine (1999) expanded on the idea of a page in the memory wallet to prompt a personal care activity by suggesting the use of reminder cards for a variety of resident repetitive behaviors. For example, if the resident repeatedly asks to use the toilet, and it is known that he or she recently used the toilet and does not have a urinary tract infection, the program explains how to write an accurate but comforting message, such as, "Mary will take me to the toilet before lunch," on a card for the resident to read whenever the need to be reminded about the information arises. To date, these training materials have been evaluated in comparison to a traditional lecture-style in-service for their effectiveness in conveying knowledge and engendering intent to use these skills by nursing assistants (Irvine, Bourgeois, & Ary, 2003); the performance of nursing assistants in using these reminder cards, however, has not yet been formally evaluated.

Additional data collected during the 4 years of this study were used to document the effects of memory books used during conversations on the content of the language produced by residents and CNAs. Dijkstra et al. (Dijkstra, Bourgeois, Burgio, & Allen, 2002; Dijkstra, Bourgeois, Petrie, Burgio, & Allen-Burge, 2002) reported improvements in residents' conversational coherence (both global and local coherence), and CNAs' use of facilitative discourse strategies (i.e., encouragement and cues). However, these analyses highlighted the fact that CNAs may require more specific training on how best to facilitate interactions with the more impaired residents with whom they tended to use a high rate of questions instead of encouragement and cues (Dijkstra et al., 2002; Hoerster, Hickey, & Bourgeois, 2001). Yet, it has also been reported that memory aid use changed CNA perceptions of the resident's level of depression; staff members who had conversations with residents with memory aids appeared to be more aware of and more positive about each resident's personal life and cognitive abilities than after baseline conversations without memory aids (Bourgeois, Dijkstra, & Hickey, 2005). Much work is still needed in this area in order to learn how best to teach CNAs to understand how to adapt and modify effective communication strategies as residents' abilities change.

In the quest to find other ways that written and picture cues in the form of memory aids could facilitate and maintain functional skills in persons with dementia, Dijkstra and Bourgeois have investigated the use of written cues in tasks that address the maintenance of personal role identities. They demonstrated that persons with dementia can perform the role of teacher in situations with young children and adults in which they are instructing them to complete the steps in a recipe using a booklet illustrating those steps (e.g., a decorated gingerbread man, banana pudding, and pizza) (Dijkstra & Bourgeois, 2004). This is only one of the many more relevant memory aid treatment applications that remain to be investigated; it is hoped that this training manual will inspire other rehabilitation professionals to explore and evaluate the use of memory aids and other written cues for the many unique expressions of memory impairment that our clients display.

One final word about the use of memory aids. We have all experienced the frustration of developing interventions for clients that are initially effective, but eventually are no longer used. It may be obvious that interventions need to change along with the client; as discussed above, a memory wallet enlarged into a memory book can address the client's need for a larger font, larger pictures, and a more substantial book to manipulate. But, in addition, there is a need for appropriate training in the use of memory aids, for both the clients and their caregivers. The long-held belief that persons with dementia have learning limitations has been dispelled by Camp and his colleagues who have demonstrated repeatedly that new learning by persons with dementia is not only possible, but can be maintained over time (Camp, Bird, & Cherry, 2000). Camp has researched one technique, Spaced Retrieval, extensively, and in comparison with other cueing hierarchy strategies (Bourgeois et al., 2003). Clients with dementia who are asked to recall specific information repeatedly over increasingly longer periods of time learn and retain this information for 4 weeks and longer (Bourgeois et al., 2003; Brush & Camp, 1998a). Therefore, training clients to use memory aids needs to be an integral part of their treatment goal [see Brush & Camp (1998b) for the details of a Spaced Retrieval training program]. Similarly, training caregivers, both family and professional, to implement procedures to practice the use of memory aids and to modify the aid as clients' needs change is needed. Camp (2005) is in the process of developing and evaluating an Internet-based Spaced Retrieval training program that complements the "Train the Trainer" in-service training program for rehabilitation professionals (Malone, Camp, & Rose, 2003).

# CHAPTER 2

# Using Memory Aids to Enhance Conversation

Think of the memory aid as a prosthetic device to help the individual to remember better—like eyeglasses help people to see better, hearing aids help to hear better, canes to walk better, and dentures to eat better. Glasses, hearing aids, canes, and dentures provide valuable assistance with basic life functions (seeing, hearing, walking, and eating) that are essential for maintaining a satisfactory quality of life. When an individual no longer benefits from these devices because of profound illness, he or she loses the ability to control his or her own quality of life and is sentenced to a life of dependency on others. Losing the ability to remember names, words, and facts forces the memory-impaired individual to rely on others in many situations. In a conversation, the person may not remember his daughter's name and has to hope that he has said enough about her that his conversational partner will know who he is talking about. He may rely on his spouse to fill in the appropriate names and words when he stumbles on them. He must depend on others to know that when the facts are not quite right he is not lying or trying to confuse his listener. He simply cannot remember the things he wants to say.

With a memory aid, the memory-impaired individual can function independently. She can keep the memory aid in her purse, pulling it out when she wants to talk with someone or when her thoughts are jumbled. Persons have been observed to keep their memory aid in a shirt pocket, or attached to a keychain on a belt loop. They spend time looking through the memory aid; family members have commented that they appear to be studying them, rehearsing the names, dates, and other facts. Others exhibit genuine pride in sharing their memory aid with other patients or staff at nursing homes and adult day centers; very animated conversations often result.

## Making Memory Wallets and Memory Books

The **memory wallet** is a collection of sentence and picture stimuli which are designed to prompt recall of the stated facts and other related factual information. The memory wallet consists of a wallet-type cover and approximately 20–30 index card (3 × 5–inch) pages on which one sentence and corresponding picture are affixed. The wallet and pages are two-hole punched and assembled with 1-inch metal rings; the pages can be laminated if desired. Alternatively, one can purchase a pocket-sized photo album with clear plastic sleeves into which the illustrated pages can be inserted. The memory wallet can be organized chronologically beginning with the birth date or organized into topics using tab inserts to denote each topic. The sentences in the memory wallet can either be typed in large print or hand printed in a bold, simple print style. The best pictures to include are those that clearly represent the stated fact, that show one or a couple (at most) people, and that are enlarged or reduced to fit the space available in the wallet.

The **memory book** is an enlarged version of the memory wallet. The cover is a 3-ring binder, and the pages are regular 8½ × 11–inch sheets of paper on which large size lettering is used to print the sentence stimuli. To protect the pages and the pictures and to provide additional weight and texture to the pages, each page can be inserted into a plastic page protector. Photo albums that have clear, magnetic pages or plastic sleeves into which completed pages can be inserted are useful too. Tabs can be used to divide the pages into different topics, as desired.

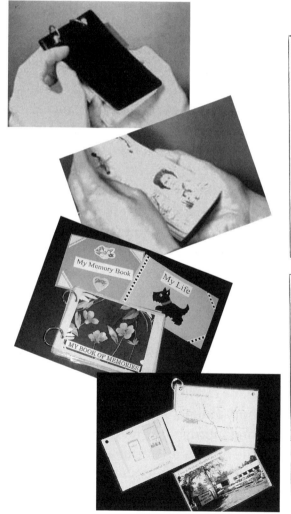

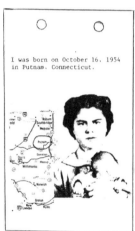

I was born on October 16, 1954 in Putnam, Connecticut.

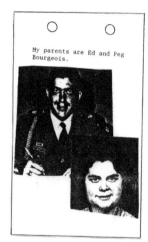

My parents are Ed and Peg Bourgeois.

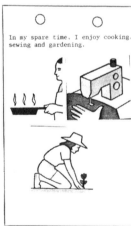

In my spare time, I enjoy cooking, sewing and gardening.

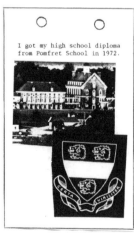

I got my high school diploma from Pomfret School in 1972.

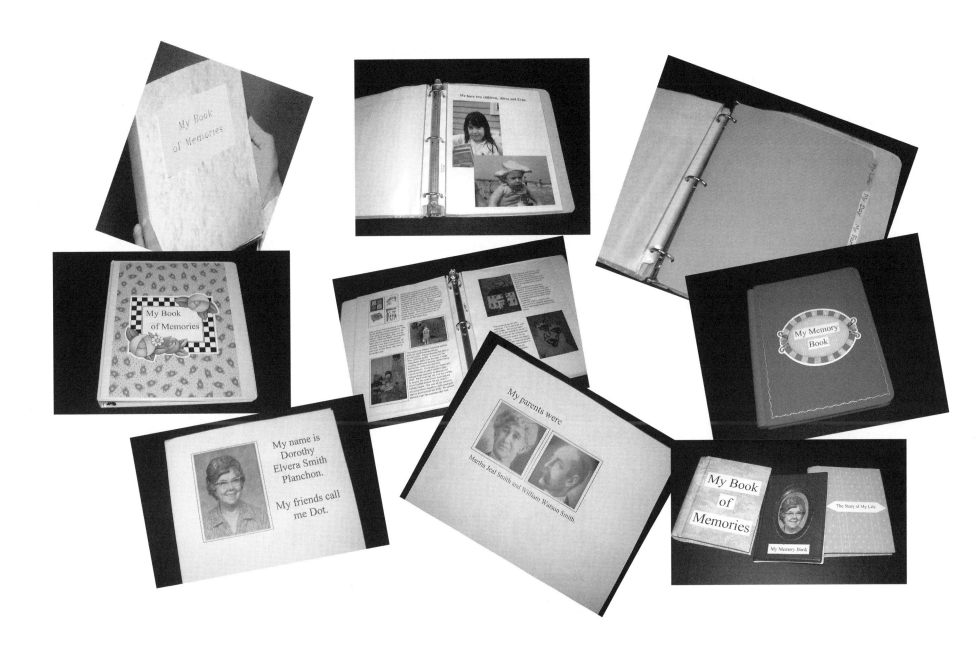

## Determining the Format

When deciding to make a memory aid, its size, format, and number of pages should be determined by the client's needs and desired function. A single page with one sentence and picture or an album illustrating 80+ years of a lifetime can provide the information needed in different circumstances.

The larger formatted memory book is useful for persons who intend to use it in their room, on a table top, or on a wheelchair tray. The larger format allows for larger print font and pictures. The disadvantage of the larger book is that it may be too heavy to carry outside the person's room or home. The memory wallet format is portable, lighter in weight, and can be attached to a walker or wheelchair (see Appendix A for ideas for transporting memory wallets). The range of font sizes that can be used with a memory wallet may be limited somewhat to smaller fonts or fewer words.

## Determining the Size of the Type

The easiest way to determine the appropriate size of the font for the printed text is to have examples of sentences in various font sizes for your client to read aloud. Notice the ease or difficulty with which your client reads the sentences; notice any self-corrections and other reading behaviors displayed by the reader. If the person comments on the content of the sentence, then there is evidence of comprehension; if the person reads with great effort or makes reading errors, a larger font size should be tried.

A useful assessment tool to construct for this purpose is a mock memory aid. The *Bourgeois Oral Reading Screen* can be copied and assembled into a five-page memory book of various sizes for this purpose.

**Examples of font sizes.**

Font Size 12
Font Size 16
Font Size 18
Font Size 20
Font Size 22
Font Size 24
Font Size 26
Font Size 28
Font Size 36
Font Size 48
Font Size 72

**Bourgeois Oral Reading Screen**
[Reprinted from Bourgeois, M. (1992). *Enhancing the conversations of memory-impaired persons: A memory aid workbook.* Gaylord, MI: Northern Speech Services, Inc.]

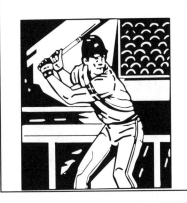

I enjoy baseball games.

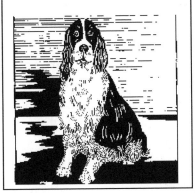

The dog's name is Rover.

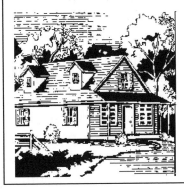

I live in Swissvale.

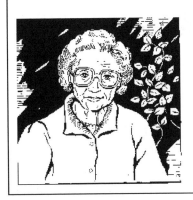

My sister is 75 years old.

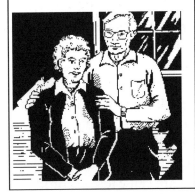

My wife's name is Mary.

## Choosing the Information for the Memory Aid

The information chosen for the aid must be facts that are important to the client, that he or she wants to talk about, and that he or she often gets confused. The memory aid should also contain facts that are important to the caregiver, such as activities of daily living and common topics of conversation. Several forms for gathering pertinent information from family or staff informants are included in Appendix C1 and C2.

Some examples of useful information to include in memory aids:

**Biography:** I was born on May 10, 1905 in Liverpool, Maryland.
My parents were Howard and Sylvia Smith.
I graduated from Liverpool High School in 1922.

**Family:** My husband is Fredrick Johnson.
Fred and I had four children.
Elena is our oldest daughter.

**Daily Life:** I wake up around 7:00 a.m. daily.
I get dressed before breakfast.
I go shopping with Fred on Tuesdays.

Nursing home or assisted living residents may not have family available to provide information and pictures, but memory aids can include information about other topics important to the resident, such as:

| People I live with: | My roommate's name is Helen Cargill. |
| | I sit next to Jane Smedley at lunch. |
| | I go to Bingo with Sam Samuels. |
| People who work here: | My favorite day nurse is Jan Friendly. |
| | The hairdresser, Arlene, curls my hair. |
| | Rev. Jones gives a good sermon on Sundays. |
| Daily schedule: | After breakfast I go to the activities room. |
| | On Monday evenings we usually see a movie. |
| | Terry comes on Wednesdays with the puppy. |

## Writing the Sentences

Persons with dementia usually demonstrate relatively preserved reading skills, although not necessarily at the same level as prior to their illness. To maximize reading success, do the following:

- **Keep the sentences short.** In the early stages of memory loss, reading a 12- to 15-word sentence may not be a problem. But in the later stages, the beginning of the sentence may be forgotten by the time the end is read. Try to limit the length to 8–10 words; even shorter is better, especially for residents who may best respond to short phrases or a couple of words, such as "my husband Jim" or "my wedding day."

- **Keep the sentence structure simple.** Simple declarative sentence structure (i.e., sentences using the verb *to be* or *to have*) seems to facilitate reading: "This is my daughter Mary"; "I have three sons, Mike, John, and Frank." Avoid using relative or dependent clauses: "I go to church on Sunday" is easier than "When it's Sunday, I go to church."

- **Use the person's vocabulary.** Compose sentences that reflect the way the person would say them. If possible, include the client in the process of making the memory aid so that his or her own words and descriptions of the pictures can be elicited. Specific words or favorite phrases can prompt familiar memories and additional elaboration. In contrast, unfamiliar vocabulary or sentence structure can cause reading

challenges; if the person is struggling to read the sentence, it will not serve the purpose of triggering related memories to discuss. The time spent planning and previewing sentences and pictures can prevent the need to make changes in a finished memory aid. It is recommended that you type out the list of memory aid sentences and ask the person to read them aloud before printing the pages to be illustrated. Any necessary changes in wording and size of font can be made before the final assembly of the memory aid.

## Illustrating the Memory Aid

You may be guided in your choice of information by the pictures that are available to go along with the text. Remember, however, that when family pictures are not available, there are ways to illustrate important facts using clip art, magazine pictures, line drawings, and other memorabilia. The following guidelines are helpful for choosing appropriate pictures:

- **Choose simple pictures.** Pictures that clearly illustrate the statement are usually pictures of a single person or object. Groups of people are difficult to label (if necessary, type small labels under each person's picture for clarity).

Pictures of an individual's head or torso may be clearer than whole body shots.

- **Adjust the size of the picture.** Copying machines have enlarging and reducing features that adjust the size of available pictures to fit the page.
- **Use copies of photographs.** Families may be reluctant to share valuable old photographs for the memory aids because they fear they will get lost or destroyed. Reassure them that all photos will be copied on a copy machine and originals will be returned. For especially valuable pictures, the family may want to do the copying themselves at their local self-service copy center. You will also want to make duplicates of all the photos in the event the memory aid gets lost or if you want to make another aid in a different format.
- **Use commercial pictures or drawings.** Photographs may not be available for all statements chosen for the memory aid. If you are artistic and can draw pictures representing the statements, simple pen-and-ink, black-and-white line drawings may be used. Commercial line drawings are available for purchase from dealers of speech therapy materials (see Appendix D for supply sources). Computer graphics software

and clip art from the Internet can be printed out to the appropriate size for the memory aid. Pictures cut out from magazines, particularly for common foods, articles of clothing, or holiday symbols, are another easy way to illustrate a memory aid page.

- **Take your own photos.** Sometimes the easiest way to get pictures is to take them yourself or to ask the staff at the facility to help document special events. Digital and instamatic cameras allow you to take pictures in the client's environment, of personal belongings, and of relevant activities.

## Assembling the Memory Aid

Using standard arts and crafts supplies (see box), the printed sentences (one per page), and photos, drawings, or pictures, create each page of the memory aid and assemble into an album or wallet. If possible, let the person choose the cover of the album or wallet; commercial photo albums provide a limitless selection of

---

SUPPLIES NEEDED for:

| Wallet | Memory Book |
|---|---|
| Small photo album or vinyl or heavy cardboard cover | Large photo album or 3-ring notebook binder |
| 3 × 5–inch index cards | 8½ × 11–inch pages, unlined white paper |
| Clear contact paper | Plastic page protectors |
| 1-inch metal rings | |
| 1-hole paper punch | 3-hole paper punch |

Glue, scissors, plastic tabs (optional)

patterns and styles that can be personalized as desired.

## Optional Modifications

- **Make tabbed topic pages.** You may want to divide the pages into categories using tabs. Write the topic name on the tab insert and attach the tab onto the right-hand edge of a blank index card or page. You may also want to write in large block letters the name of the topic (i.e., Family, My Life, etc.) centered on the card or page.

## Updating the Content

The advantage of this sort of memory aid is that it can be modified as events, people, and needs change. Pages are easily added whenever a significant event occurs or removed if they are no longer accurate. Encourage others to make pages for the book, or to send pictures to add to the memory aid.

When interest in the memory aid wanes, it might be time to change the format of the aid; larger print and pictures may be needed. Enlarging the existing pages is recommended, particularly for people who have enjoyed their memory wallet for a while. They may have some expectation of what picture will appear on the next page and if the stimuli had triggered a familiar story, using the same but larger stimulus should help to maintain that story. A handout for *Making Memory Aids* is included in Appendix B1.

## Using the Memory Aid in Conversation

The memory book or memory wallet is designed to be used by the individual with memory impairment as a prompt to remember a name or an event during conversations and to trigger associated and elaborated memories. The book or wallet can also be used as the focus of the conversation, to show to friends while reminiscing about their past lives. Families or staff may need to ensure that the book or wallet is available to the person—in plain view within the immediate surroundings, in a shirt or pants pocket, or in a purse before the person leaves the house—in order for it to serve its purpose in supporting conversations.

Different uses of memory aids have been observed as a function of dementia severity. In the early stages of memory loss, individuals are aware of their memory lapses. Therefore, they can participate in the development of the categories and content of their memory book. Ask them what particular words or types of words they have forgotten recently. Make sure the format of the memory book or wallet is such that they can add pages or content to the pages (i.e., do not laminate). It is not unusual for persons to make notes of related information on a page when they are reviewing their memory book alone; one individual listed the various different jobs he had held over his career with the railroad on the back of the memory wallet page that stated, "I worked for the railroad for 35 years." During conversation on the following day when he came to that page in his memory wallet he remarked, "I know you know that I worked for the railroad for 35 years, but I'll bet you didn't know that I started out in the mailroom, then I was promoted to. . . ." Another person confided that she had taken her memory wallet on a bus trip with her sisters' friends so that she could remind herself of different topics of conversation and the names of specific people and places by referring to her memory wallet when the others were not around.

Persons who present with memory losses that are not within the range of a clinical diagnosis, or preclinical, may not be ready to accept the "memory book or wallet" concept because it might appear to reflect more disability than they have or recognize yet. More naturalistic memory aids, such as daily planners and appointment books, are often more acceptable, particularly if the person had used one during his or her years of employment. It is recognized as the commonsense approach; a planner/organizer had been useful to them for remembering appointments, business associates, telephone numbers, and travel plans when they worked. It can serve a similar purpose in their retirement years. In addition to the calendar pages for tracking appointments, there can be a telephone directory, and notes pages for lists of names, categories of words, and other useful things to remember.

Individuals in the middle stages of dementia often lose awareness of the changes in their conversational behavior and that of their conversational partner. When using a memory wallet or memory book, they are often so pleased that they can participate in a conversation that they may be unaware that they are dominating the conversation or that their conversational partner may have already heard that information. In fact, some people have been observed to read aloud and elaborate about each page in their memory book, and then start over from the beginning again.

The positive view of this stage is that the person in the middle stage of dementia can be very happily occupied in the

task of telling someone else all about his or her memory book. And when his or her conversational partner is another person with dementia, it is usually not noticed by the other person that he or she has heard the same anecdote previously. In a study conducted in a nursing home, Bourgeois (1993) showed that two persons with dementia would discuss each others' memory books with several positive results, including positive reports from the nursing staff who appreciated having a positive way to engage their residents in a "normal" activity—conversation—without staff involvement.

In the late stages of dementia, individuals' cognitive decline may be expressed as reduced verbal output, apparent lack of interest in visual stimuli, and self-stimulatory behavior such as repetitive vocalization, tactile exploration, and repetitive movements (e.g., rocking, hit-

ting, pacing). When presented with a memory wallet or memory book, this person may not use it independently to read aloud the printed statements or elaborate on the topic. The physical characteristics of the aid may need to be altered for it to be a useful prompting system; there may need to be larger pages and font size, or the sentences may need to be simpler in syntactic complexity. The subject of the memory book may need to be something highly interesting to the person, such as a hobby or sport; interest albums can be a useful activity for the person who has limited capacity to engage in group activities. Once the appropriate memory aid is determined, it will be the caregiver's job to make sure it is within reach, to assist with turning the pages, and to provide a narration of the memory aid if it does not elicit any coherent output. Confused utterances may make some sense if there

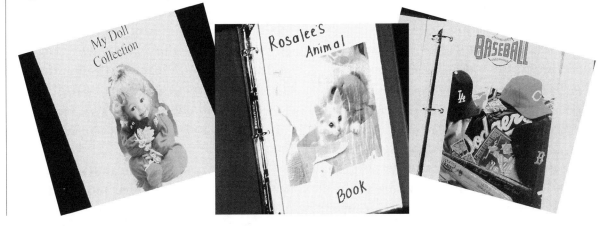

is a referent on the page. Changes in affect, or nonverbal communication (i.e., a smile, a frown, increased rate of breathing, straighter posture, etc.), may signal recognition of the stimulus on the page.

The amount of vigilance of the wallets/books required by caregivers seems to be related to the cognitive abilities of the client. In the early stages of memory loss, individuals are usually very aware of their memory problems and of the usefulness of the memory aid. Therefore, mildly memory-impaired individuals are usually pretty good at keeping the memory aid with them, putting it someplace sensible, and remembering to use it when they need to. Moderately memory-impaired persons have little trouble using the memory aid when it is on the table in front of them, in their pocket or purse, or handed to them by the caregiver; but, if it is not in plain view, they may not remember to look for it or to ask someone to help them find it. At this stage, caregivers have to increase their own attention to the wallet/book, ensuring that it remains in an obvious and accessible place. It may be helpful to have a designated place to keep the wallet/book (i.e., on the kitchen table, on the coffee table in the TV room, by the telephone, etc.) so that the memory-impaired individual can learn to expect to find it in

that same place and can put it back there when he or she is finished with it. Some persons carry their memory wallet on an expandable key chain from a belt loop; others tolerate hanging it around their neck on a lanyard. The sensation of the wallet banging against a leg or dangling near the stomach prompts persons to look through the wallet periodically. Handing the memory aid to the person, and saying "Read this," or pointing to it when a specific problem occurs, instead of responding with a verbal explanation, can be quite successful. Caregivers have reported success at reducing repetitive questions and behaviors, including sundowning, by having the person read the accurate information in the memory aid.

Day care and nursing staff have found the memory aids a useful tool for redirecting restless clients to converse with another person. People who wander around a facility, approaching staff with repetitive requests to call family members or to leave the facility, can be encouraged to show their wallet/book to someone else, thereby interrupting the disruptive behavior. Staff are then able to complete other duties and return to converse with the client at another time.

The memory aids can be particularly useful for unfamiliar conversational partners, such as volunteers in a nursing

home, who may want to engage the memory-impaired person in conversation but have difficulty because the person is very confused, cannot maintain a conversational topic, or is unintelligible. The book/wallet can help the volunteer to talk and ask specific questions about the pictures, reading the sentence prompts for accuracy. Volunteers have expressed their satisfaction with the memory books/wallets because they feel they are helping the individual to talk about important people and events in his or her life when they use it and to talk more accurately and with less confusion. For the volunteer who may feel uncomfortable thinking of ways to interact with the memory-impaired person, the memory book/wallet provides a concrete activity in which to engage. Nursing staff have been observed to initiate conversation with a resident when the memory book is on the table in front of the resident and to remark that they had no idea the resident looked so beautiful in her youth, or had had such an interesting life or so many children. The memory book provides humanizing information for the caregivers about residents who require so much physical care that the caregivers do not have time to become familiar with the details of their clients' personal lives.

## Getting the Conversation Started and Keeping It Going

Starting the conversation in a positive way helps people with memory impairment feel comfortable talking and minimizes the frustration of forgetting what they want to tell you.

You do this by:

1. *Asking* them to have a conversation with you.

   > "Mary, I'd really like to talk with you today. Would you mind if I sat down beside you?"

   By asking them to have the conversation with you, you are letting them know that you value their friendship and that you feel they are worth talking with. You are also giving them a sense of control over their lives; instead of always being required to do what is scheduled next for them, they can agree, or not, to spend the next few minutes of their day talking with you. Most often these individuals will be overjoyed to break the routine by conversing with you, to be given the opportunity to share some thoughts or anxieties. Ending the conversation can be the most difficult aspect of these interactions; although if you have had a satisfying conversation because of the memory aid, you can sincerely reassure them that you would enjoy coming back to talk with them, if they would like that, of course.

2. *Guiding* the conversation onto specific topics and *redirecting* the conversation back to the topic when the person begins to ramble keeps the conversation going.

   > "Mary, let's talk about your family first, please tell me all about them."

   > "That's very interesting, and what else do you do during the day, Bob?"

   Although many memory-impaired individuals will know what they want to talk about and will do so without prompting, they do tend to forget some of the common conversational manners/courtesies (such as, not taking too long of a turn, talking about the same thing repeatedly, or switching the topic too soon). You may need to guide the conversation onto specific topics that you are also interested in talking about, to change the topic when there's nothing more new to say about the current one, or to ask follow-up questions about a topic that was changed too quickly. You can do this gently, in a nonconfrontational manner, by assuring the person that you are interested in what he or she is saying (with a smile, a nod, or a word like "good," "interesting," or "OK"), and then interjecting a comment or question, for example, "Good, now tell me what else Mary did last night after dinner." If a subtle redirection is not effective, a more direct approach can be used: "I understand your concern about the dishes, we'll talk some more about that later; now let's talk about what we'll need to take on our trip."

3. *Reassuring* the person and *helping out* when he or she gets stuck or can't find the right word to use.

   > "That's OK, Bob; what else can you tell me about your life?"

   > "I think Market Square is where you bought that delicious fish, right?"

   All of us lose a word here or there in the course of a story we are telling, and it can be both frustrating and embarrassing. Fortunately for us, we can usually retrieve the word quickly and continue on with our discourse. The memory-impaired person, however, may spend a long time trying to find the word and in the end not find it at all. The most helpful strategy is to provide the word if you know it so that the conversation can continue. Actively helping the person with a word reassures him or her that what he or she has to say is important to you.

4. *Smiling* and *acting interested* in whatever the person is talking about even if you are not quite sure what the person is trying to say. The desire to communicate is innately human. Most people, even those severely confused, retain the primitive need to connect with others. Even if verbal communication no longer makes sense, the nonverbal behaviors of conversational partners can serve to reassure the person that he or she still belongs in the speaking world. A smile and a nod says you value the person and what it is he or she is attempting to say.

5. *Thanking* the person for talking with you. A word of thanks at the end of the conversation conveys your appreciation for the person's willingness to talk with you. It implies that he or she was in control of the conversation; that it would not have occurred without the person's permission. This feeling of control, of independence, can be rare if the person is in a situation in which he or she has to depend on others for so many other aspects of daily living. Thanking the person is also a useful transition device; it may be difficult to end a conversation and move on to the next activity. Interrupting the conversation with a gentle word of thanks is often very effective in ending the conversational topic and getting the person to anticipate the next activity. A handout of these instructions, *Guidelines for Having a Satisfying Conversation,* is included as Appendix B2.

## What to AVOID During Conversations

• *DO NOT Quiz* the person or ask lots of specific questions, such as

"Now who is this person? I know you know who it is?"

"Are you sure that's Mary? I thought it was Barbara."

Quizzing the person puts him or her on the spot and produces nervous and anxious feelings. If the person is not offering much information, your job is to do the talking; start a topic of conversation with a statement like, "I was remembering that day Mary cornered the gator in the backyard, wasn't that scary?"

• *DO NOT Correct* or *contradict* something that was stated as a fact even if you know it is wrong.

"No, that's not John. That's Jason, remember, your grandson Jason?"

Correcting and contradicting someone is demeaning, making the person feel childish and argumentative, and stifling any desires for future conversational interactions. A subtle, positive, and effective way of communicating the accurate information is to restate the statement with the correct information: "Jason does look a lot like John, doesn't he?"

## Troubleshooting

What if . . .

1. **They lose the memory aid?**

   • Make a copy of the pages before you give it to them.
   • Decide on a dedicated location and keep the memory aid there.
   • Label the location: "My memory book stays here."
   • Attach the aid to them (see Appendix A for wearable devices: necklace, vest pocket, apron, belt, wristband)
   • Attach the aid to walker or wheelchair (see Appendix A for walker/wheelchair bags)

- Identify typical hiding places for personal valuables (underwear drawer, closet)

2. **They do not want to use the memory aid?**

   - Embarrassed to use it—Modify a monthly planner.
   - Difficulty seeing print—Modify font size, convert wallet to book format.

3. **They have reading problems?**

   - Cannot see the words—Change print font; check for eyeglasses.
   - Substitute words—Consider revising the sentence with their words.
   - Make reading errors—Simplify text and enlarge font size.

- Substitute nonwords—Restate sentence as written.
- Read slowly—May need to enlarge print, shorten sentences.
- Omit words—Simplify and enlarge text.

4. **They have difficulty turning the pages?**

   - May need to switch to larger format.
   - May need to strengthen pages with lamination or plastic page protectors.
   - Remove pages from book, present them one at a time within visual field.
   - Remove pages from wallet, encourage card-dealing motion.
   - Turn pages for person.

5. **They argue with written statements?**

   - Change wording to their wording.
   - Ask them to describe a picture, then use their words to change statement.
   - Remove page from aid.

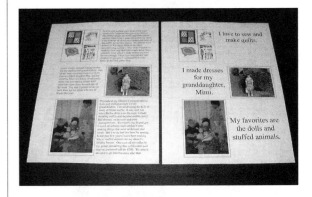

**Example of modifying a memory book when the text becomes too small to read.**

Sample Memory Book (*continued on following page*)

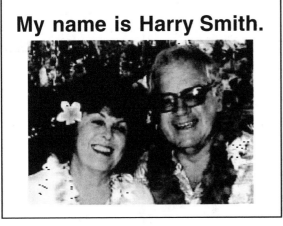

**My name is Harry Smith.**

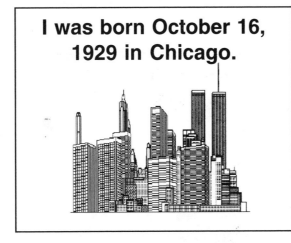

**I was born October 16, 1929 in Chicago.**

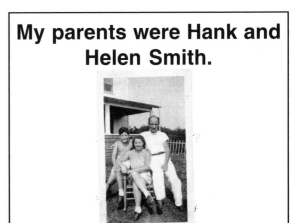

**My parents were Hank and Helen Smith.**

I have one grandchild.
Her name is Hillary.

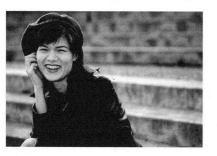

I enjoy traveling.

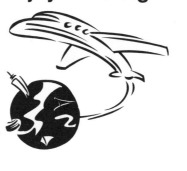

I also love to read.

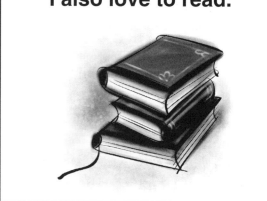

I live at Oak Park.

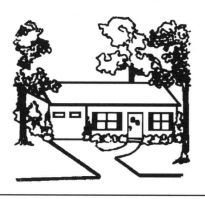

Cindy is my day-time nurse.

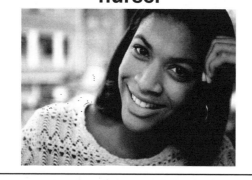

Lunch is served at 12:15.

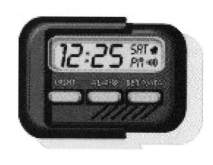

Eating keeps me strong and healthy.

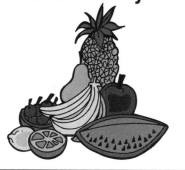

Showers help me feel fresh and clean.

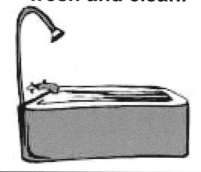

A good night's rest gives me energy.

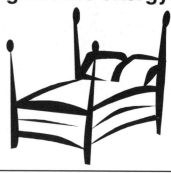

# CHAPTER 3

# Using Memory Aids to Enhance Orientation

## Information Needs Assessment

Orientation to person, place, and time is often impaired as a result of neurological conditions. Problems in recall and recognition of personal knowledge and self-identity can create fear and confusion. Luckily, these problems can be addressed using a variety of memory aids in written and picture formats for persons at different stages of impaired cognition and for different treatment settings (home/community, assisted living/nursing home, hospital). Standard and informal assessment techniques will yield specific deficits requiring memory supports. For example, the *Mini-Mental State Exam* (MMSE) (Folstein, Folstein, & McHugh, 1975) includes 10 orientation questions (e.g., What is the day, date, month, year, season? Where are we now, street address, city, state, county?). Many other assessment tools include orientation questions that are helpful in developing treatment goals. It must be noted, however, that the assessed deficits in orientation skills may not always suggest functional treatment goals; in fact, the opposite is often observed in clinical settings. For example, clinicians may determine that the client does not respond accurately to standard questions about day, date, year, and season and develop a treatment goal to address this specific deficit. The client may "learn" to obtain the correct answers to orientation questions from a therapy task involving a monthly calendar page in the treatment room, but not transfer this learning to the home environment where there may not be a similarly formatted calendar or the opportunity to answer orientation questions as queried by the clinician. This failure to generalize from the clinical to the home setting could be avoided by designing orientation-related therapy tasks that address the client-specific functional applications of those skills in the desired locations. This requires knowledge of the desired post-therapy behaviors prior to developing the treatment plan. Therefore, a critical component of assessment would be the client, family, and caregiver interview to determine the types and complexity of orientation skills that were used before the memory impairment and those needed for maintaining the quality of life expected or desired after the memory loss. The Orientation Assessment Form (Appendix C3) can be used to obtain the necessary information to guide functional treatment goal selection.

For example, the retired lawyer who is now challenged by early signs of dementia and admits to some recent missed appointments and disorientation on occasion when driving would benefit from an assessment of what tools he has used in the past to keep oriented. It is likely that he used multiple tools while he was employed, including the electronic calendar on his desktop computer and his personal digital assistant (PDA), programming each to signal upcoming appointments. Now that he is retired, he has relaxed his attitude about keeping organized and only enters information into his PDA on occasion. Similarly, he may have depended on the Global Posi-

tioning System (GPS) feature of his automobile when traveling around the state for work, but does not acknowledge the potential utility of the GPS for familiar locations around town. A couple of simple modifications to the systems he has already used successfully should enable him to maintain his desired level of independence during this period of his life, such as deciding to use one calendar system (the PDA) on a daily basis and using the GPS for around town driving. As the memory impairment increases, these tools can be further modified to maintain orientation to person (by using written identity supports), to place (by using written place supports such as driving directions), and to time (by switching to written planners, then wall calendars).

It is important to acknowledge that this functional approach to orientation behaviors focuses on the effective use of compensatory strategies to achieve a desired state or accomplish a desired task with the orientation information, and *not* the simple recitation of this information. One cannot assume that a person can use the information stated in a therapy task for a real-life situation or that it would even be relevant to another situa-

tion. For example, if the client learns to state, "I am in the hospital," in response to the question, "Where are you now?" there is no reason to trust that that same question will elicit the correct information when he returns home and has to state his address to the emergency operator on the phone. Instead of teaching specific orientation facts, there would be an increased likelihood of generalization if therapy focused on teaching an orientation strategy—when you want to know where you are, refer to the written location information. The hospitalized patient could be instructed to read the orientation facts written on a message board (see tabletop message board on page 32) and the family could be instructed to display a similar message board at home with the relevant information. Similarly, the nursing home resident should be instructed to read the correct information from his or her memory book or the orientation board when that information needs to be accessed. Therefore, the following examples of written supports for orientation behaviors are meant to be used in the development of compensatory strategies for orientation *behaviors* and not the relearning of orientation *facts*.

## Sample Orientation Assessment Form (Appendix C3)

| Past Behaviors for location/profession: Retired Lawyer | | Desired Behaviors for location/activities: home, drives to golf course, doctors, and church | |
|---|---|---|---|
| **Person:** Oriented to person | **Supports:** Driver's license | **Person:** Needs personal identity information | **Supports:** Driver's license<br>Wallet identity card |
| **Place:** Oriented to place | Used maps some<br>Used GPS in car | **Place:** Needs written location information for emergency use<br>Needs written supports for directions to familiar locations | Written address by telephone & in wallet<br>Driving directions notebook for car |
| **Time:** Oriented to time | Wristwatch<br>Electronic calendar on computer<br>PDA<br>Cell phone | **Time:** Needs to keep daily appointments<br>Worried about taxes & bill paying | Consolidate electronic systems (computer, PDA, or cell phone)<br>Use monthly wall calendar to note bill/tax due dates<br>Wristwatch |

## Memory Aid Examples

# Orientation to Person (Personal Knowledge, Identity)

1. Personal identification card in wallet, purse, or planner

2. Medic Alert necklace or bracelet

---

Name:        Melissa Browning
Address:     1234 Ivy Street
             My City, My State, Zipcode
Telephone:   (555) 123-4567
In case of emergency:
        Notify: Harvey Browning, my brother
        Telephone:   (555) 234-5678
Medical Alert: Allergic to penicillin
My doctor is:  Dr. William Smith at St. Mary's Hospital
             Telephone: (555) 567-8912

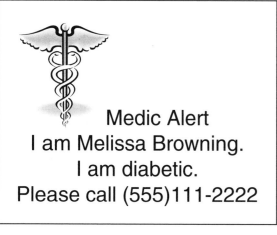

Medic Alert
I am Melissa Browning.
I am diabetic.
Please call (555)111-2222

3. Name tags

| My Name is |
| --- |
| Melissa Browning |

4. To enhance self-recognition, place labeled self-photo in relevant location (e.g., on mirror if she thinks the person in the mirror is a stranger).

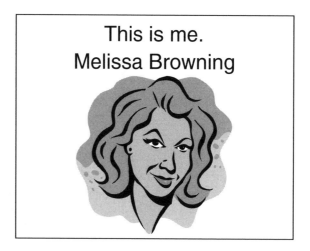

This is me.
Melissa Browning

5. To enhance self-recognition, place labeled past and current self-photos in memory book.

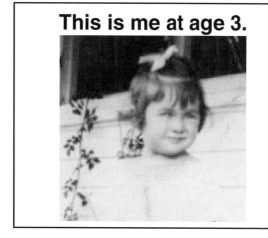

This is me at age 3.

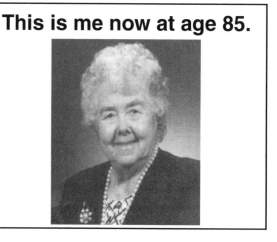

This is me now at age 85.

## Orientation to Place: Physical Location (Immediate, Residence, Community)

1. Immediate location

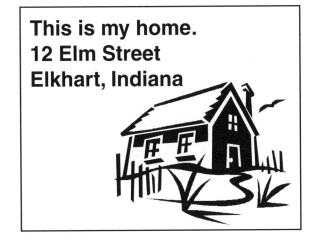

**This is my home.**
**12 Elm Street**
**Elkhart, Indiana**

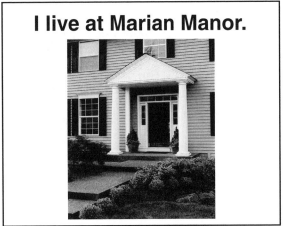

**I live at Marian Manor.**

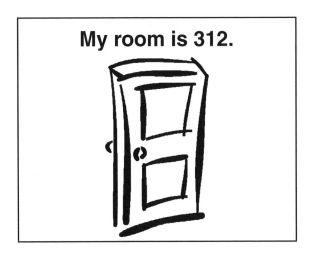

**My room is 312.**

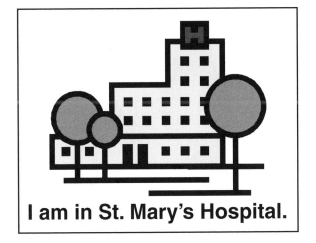

**I am in St. Mary's Hospital.**

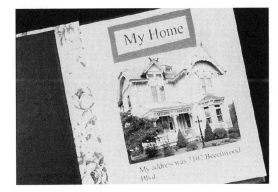

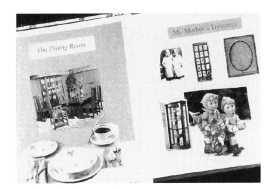

2. Community locations

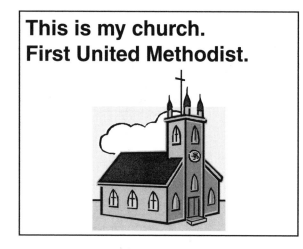

This is my church.
First United Methodist.

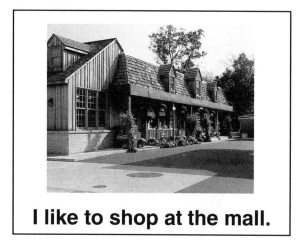

I like to shop at the mall.

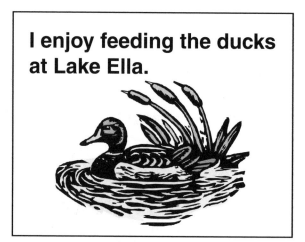

I enjoy feeding the ducks at Lake Ella.

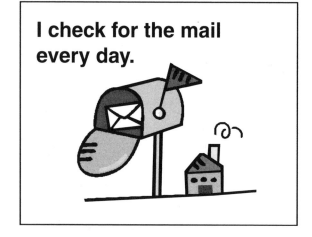

I check for the mail every day.

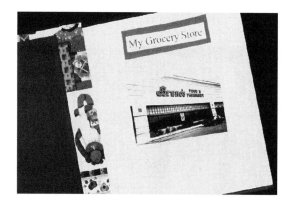

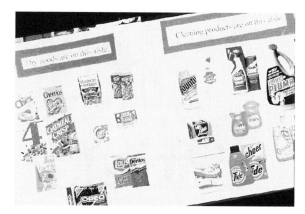

3.  Within specific locations: Grocery store

**Shopping Lists by Food Category and by Store Route**

| Shopping List | |
|---|---|
| **Dairy** | Milk, yogurt, cheese |
| **Meats** | Hamburger, chicken breast |
| **Vegetables** | Carrots, lettuce, celery |
| **Canned Goods** | Baked beans, pasta, coffee |
| **Frozen Foods** | Ice cream |
| **Paper goods** | Paper napkins, toilet paper |
| **Cleaning** | Sponge, detergent |
| | |

**Driving Instructions**
**(to be included in a driving notebook)**

**From Home to Grocery Store**

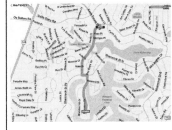

1.  **Turn RIGHT at end of driveway.**
2.  **Turn LEFT at stop sign (Shamrock Rd.)**
3.  **Turn RIGHT at Shannon Lakes Rd.**
4.  **Turn LEFT at shopping center entrance**
5.  **Park the car.**

**From Grocery Store to Home**

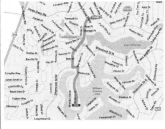

1.  **Drive to shopping center entrance.**
2.  **Turn RIGHT onto Shannon Lakes Rd.**
3.  **Turn LEFT at stop sign (Shamrock Rd).**
4.  **Turn RIGHT at Edenderry Drive.**
5.  **Turn LEFT into home driveway.**

4. Hospital: Acute care

a. Tabletop message board (clear plastic frame with laminated messages)

b. For nurse

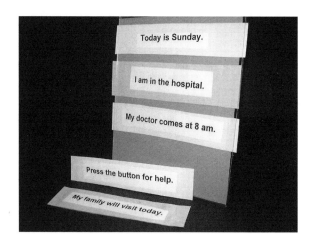

| Today is: | Monday, June 4, 2006 |
|---|---|
| ■ | I'm in the hospital. |
| ■ | I've had a stroke/accident. |
| ■ | I'm going to X-ray. |
| ■ | I'm going to rehab. |
| ■ | I'm going to the doctor. |
| ■ | My family knows I'm here. |
| ■ | My family is coming later. |

| | |
|---|---|
| ■ | I am your nurse. |
| ■ | This is your water glass. |
| ■ | You have a catheter. |
| ■ | Press the button to call me. |
| ■ | Don't try to get up alone. |

| I'm here to: |
|---|
| ■ take your blood pressure |
| ■ take your temperature |
| ■ draw blood |
| ■ give you a bath/shower |
| ■ change your dressing |
| ■ change your bed |
| ■ get you dressed |
| ■ give you medicine |
| ■ get you out of bed |

# Orientation to Time

1. Watches and clocks

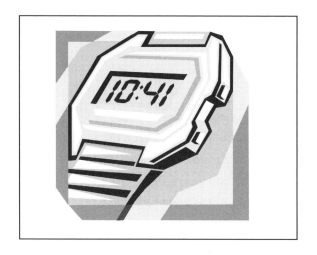

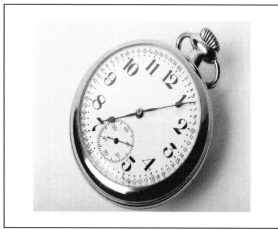

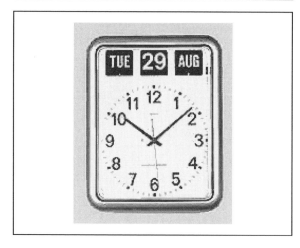

2. Planners and calendars (monthly, weekly, daily)

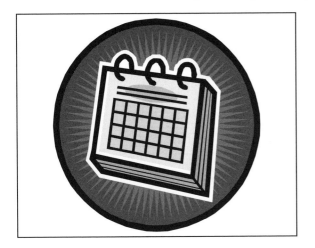

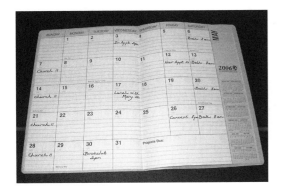

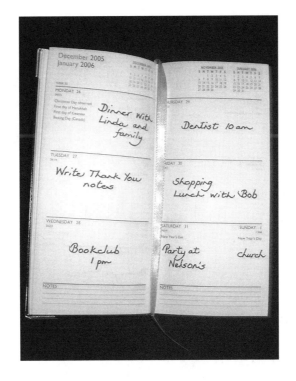

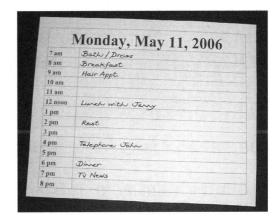

3. Reminder cards

| | |
|---|---|
| **If I want to know what day it is, I look at the calendar.** 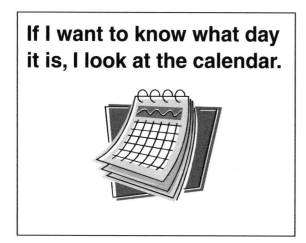 | **If I want to know what time it is, I look at the clock.** 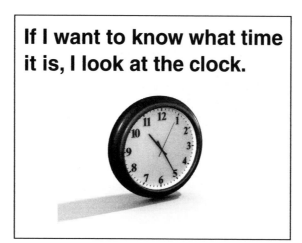 |

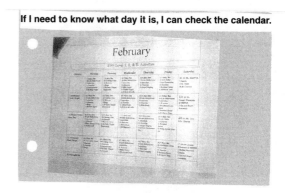

If I need to know what day it is, I can check the calendar.

4. Reality orientation boards

| **Today is** | Saturday, April 14 |
|---|---|
| **The year is** | 2006 |
| **The season is** | Spring |
| **The next holiday is** | Easter and Passover |
| **This is** | St. Mary's Residence |
| **The city is** | Providence |
| **The state is** | New Jersey |
| **The weather is** | Sunny and warm ☼ |

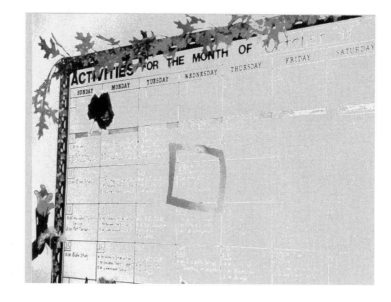

# CHAPTER 4

# Using Memory Aids to Enhance Communication of Wants, Needs, and Safety

## Information Needs and Environmental Assessment

The most fundamental purpose of communication may well be to convey personal desires and preferences; to express the need for interaction, engagement, intimacy, satisfaction of hunger, thirst, and comfort; and to prevent harm to oneself or others. When the necessary words to express these ideas are limited by memory impairment, it is important to provide supports that the individual can use to convey the accurate message.

In the home environment, family caregivers may be particularly knowledgeable about the personal preferences of their family members and be able to accommodate their desires without much overt communication. When this person moves to a residential facility, however, he or she may need to have some means of sharing this knowledge with the new caregivers. Memory books, and other written supports with the relevant information, can provide a clear and direct way for the person to indicate what he or she would like or needs.

This chapter provides ideas for a variety of specific cues and cuing formats for communicating personally relevant information. The examples below include common exemplars in the categories of wants (personal preferences), needs, and safety in a variety of settings; each individual will have his or her own unique needs that will require creative adaptations of these suggestions. Interviewing the client, the family, and caregivers will yield the most appropriate and useful personal messages. The Personal Wants, Needs, and Safety Assessment Form (Appendix C4) can be completed to obtain relevant information for treatment planning and for a successful transition from one living arrangement to another. Some residential facilities have family members complete a social history form about the client before relocation so that staff members can incorporate some personal information into their initial interactions with the client in order to be welcoming and to convey a sense of familiarity. Personal possessions to decorate the new room will create a sense of home; staff members who talk about the resident's family and favorite activities will seem like old friends.

The suggestions in this chapter can be used with the client as a means for him or her to communicate to others specific wants and needs, or as a way for him or her to use cues to remember specific information, details, or sequences that will enable optimal independence in functioning. For example, the resident with moderate to severe dementia moving into the nursing home may need to have a memory book with a specific section on personal preferences. The nursing staff can read it to learn that she likes her bath before bed, her coffee black, and her radio tuned in to the classical channel. This same memory book can have a section that she can use to follow for the correct sequence for getting dressed by herself, or to remember what activities are offered on which days at this facility. If this person is ambulatory, a portable memory book should include pages that

remind her where her room is located, what activities she enjoys, and when meals are scheduled. She should have this book attached to her in a comfortable way such that she can refer to it whenever she needs to or so that staff can show her where to find the answers to her questions in her book. The postsurgical patient with cognitive impairment due to the effects of anesthesia may need visual supports for communicating the need for pain medication or other comfort measures; an emotions page in a memory book, a tabletop message board, or a picture card pain assessment tool can be useful to patients and nurses who need to document patient status periodically.

Safety concerns can place the person with memory impairment at risk for more restrictions and limitations than he or she may desire; visual cues can help maintain individual independence by supporting memory for the safety strategies required by family and staff. Medication mismanagement is often one of the earliest signs of memory decline. The availability of daily and weekly pill containers with labeled compartments has helped the general public remember to take their medications as prescribed; as memory impairment increases, however, additional cues and strategies, particularly written cues, may be required to maintain

compliance. Remembering to use a walker or cane, or to ambulate safely, are challenges to those who are recovering from surgery or have frequent falls. This chapter also provides examples of a variety of picture and sentence reminder cards for these types of safety concerns.

Just as it was important for the orientation behaviors in the previous chapter to be addressed in a functional way, it is equally important for the cues and strategies developed for the communication of wants, needs, and safety to be functional. This requires knowing the personal preferences and history of the person when developing materials and training protocols, and to the extent possible, including the person in this process. Give the person choices about the content, wording, appearance, and placement of supportive cues. When people have choices they are more likely to use what they selected. For example, when this author first made wearable devices (e.g., vests, walker pockets, and lanyards; see Appendix A) for portable memory books, residents were inconsistent in using the devices. Providing a selection of devices and allowing them to choose their preferred device resulted in residents wearing and using their memory books consistently.

The degree to which the person's environment is familiar and accessible will determine the extent to which supportive cues are needed to maintain function. An unfamiliar setting, such as a nursing home or assisted living residence, will need to be assessed for the critical locations (e.g., bathroom, dining room, closet, dresser, telephone) and important activities (e.g., church services, beauty salon, gardening) in order to develop the appropriate visual supports. In the home setting, the types of necessary cues will be related to the degree to which the desired locations and activities are routine and in familiar places. If a large dry-erase calendar has been on the wall next to the phone for many years and it was consulted daily, the client may not need additional cues for it to maintain its functional use. In contrast, when this client moves to another residence, cues to the location of the calendar will need to be developed in order for this support to be accessible to the client. Similarly, if the spouse always put the newspaper by the client's plate at the breakfast table at home, to maintain the pleasure of reading the newspaper once he's moved to the assisted living facility it would be important to arrange for the paper to be put in a similar location. Alternatively, a written cue explaining where to find the newspaper could also help to maintain that activity.

## Personal Wants, Needs, and Safety Assessment Form (Appendix C4)

| | |
|---|---|
| Assessing the Wants, Needs, Safety of: | Margaret Jones (name) |
| Environment: Home Hospital (Assisted Living) Nursing Home (circle one) | |

**Wants: The expression of personal preferences, likes, and dislikes**

| Likes: | Dislikes: |
|---|---|
| Toast & black coffee for breakfast | Bright light (keep blinds semi-drawn) |
| Bath in the evening before bed | Broccoli, rutabaga, slimy foods, peppermint |
| Books, stuffed animals, a favorite shawl | Large group activities |
| Classical music; she played the violin | Frank, a former neighbor who was mean to her dog. |
| Prefers to be alone in her room. | |

**Needs: The satisfaction of physical comforts and emotional needs**

| Physical: 3-hour toilet schedule; needs minimal assistance except for supervised ambulation <br> Pain: Recovering from hip fracture (5/7/06) <br> Pain levels range from 5–7 on a good day | Emotional: <br> Likes to be touched on hands, hugged <br> Family pictures and her bible are comforting <br> Likes animals |
|---|---|

**Safety: The prevention of harm to oneself or others**

Medication: Uses 7-day pill container; needs to be on her dresser & monitored for compliance
Falls prevention: Uses 4-footed cane to ambulate; has walker for use when tired
Eating: Low tolerance for bad table manners; prefers to sit with two friends
Personal hygiene: Weekly hairdresser appointment; requires minimal monitoring in bath for safety; independent with personal grooming

**Environmental constraints:** Used to have large calendar in her kitchen to keep track of date, appointments, visitors; she will need to be reminded to monitor the RO board and her room calendar. Used to being alone; she will need to be invited to join activities.

**Emergency contacts:** Daughter, Barbara (777-888-9999) lives in Denver; works evenings and weekends. Best to call in daytime. Friend, Sally (333-444-5555) lives nearby; willing to chat on phone when she's lonely.

## Memory Aid Examples

### Wants: The Expression of Personal Preferences, Likes, and Dislikes

I prefer my bath before bedtime.

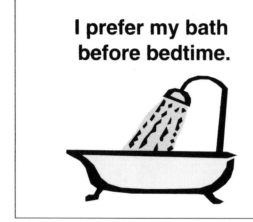

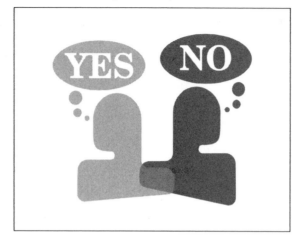

I love getting mail from my friends.

NO SMOKING, Please!

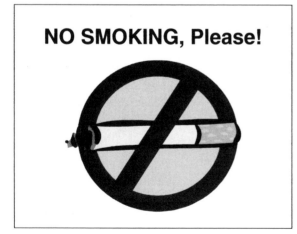

Please turn the TV OFF!

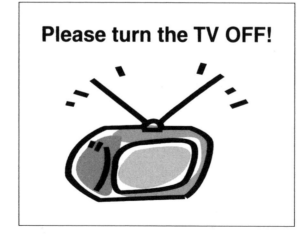

Please get my music.

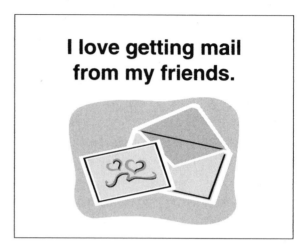

**Memory Aid Examples** (*Continued*)

**I enjoyed cooking meals for my family.**

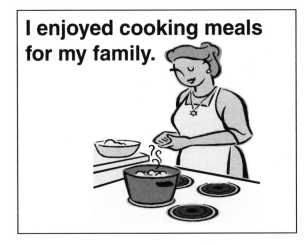

**I like salt and pepper on my food.**

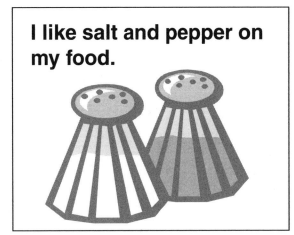

**I like teaching my granddaughter to cook.**

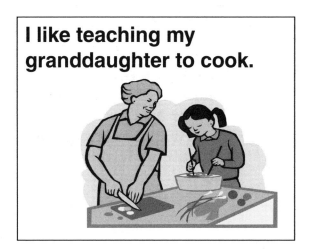

**I enjoy a steak on the grill.**

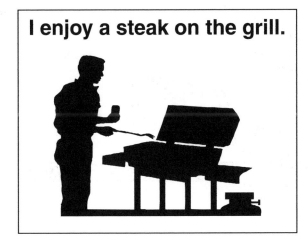

**Apple pies are my favorite.**

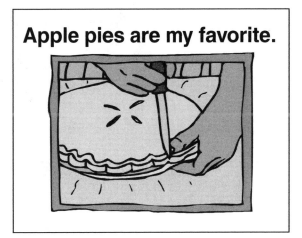

**I enjoy a glass of wine with dinner.**

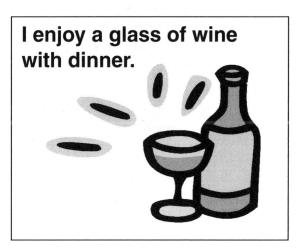

**Memory Aid Examples (*Continued*)**

| I want: | |
|---|---|
| | to sit up |
| | a blanket |
| | the TV on/off |
| | the lights on/off |
| | the blinds open/closed |
| | paper and pencil |
| | a newspaper/magazine |
| | to call my family |
| | to hold hands |
| | |

| I like: | |
|---|---|
| | my shower in the morning |
| | 2 sugars in my coffee |
| | to be alone |
| I don't like: | |
| | This music/TV show |
| | pepper |
| | Bingo |
| | |
| | |

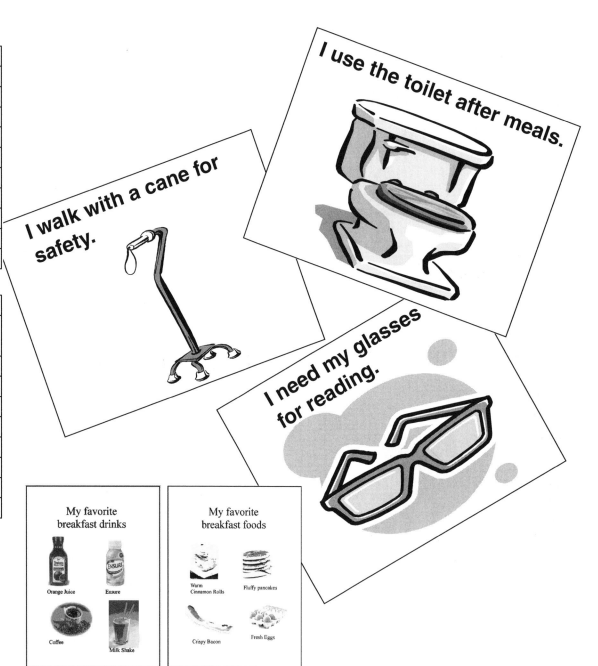

# Needs: The Satisfaction of Hunger, Thirst, Physical Comforts, Emotional Needs

Checklists:

| I Need | |
|---|---|
| | to eat |
| | to drink |
| | the bathroom |
| | pain medicine |
| | my breathing machine/inhaler |
| | my glasses |
| | my teeth |
| | my hearing aid |
| | a hug |

| *My Breakfast Selection* | |
|---|---|
| | Scrambled eggs |
| | Two eggs over easy |
| | Bacon |
| | Sausage |
| | Grapefruit |
| | Tea |
| | Coffee |
| | Sugar |
| | Creamer |
| | Toast |
| | Bagel |

Message magnets:

| |
|---|
| **I am hungry.** |
| **I am thirsty.** |
| **I am hot.** |
| **I am cold.** |
| **I am sleepy.** |
| **I am bored.** |
| **Leave me alone.** |
| **I want to pray.** |
| **I want to go outside.** |
| |

Pain assessments:

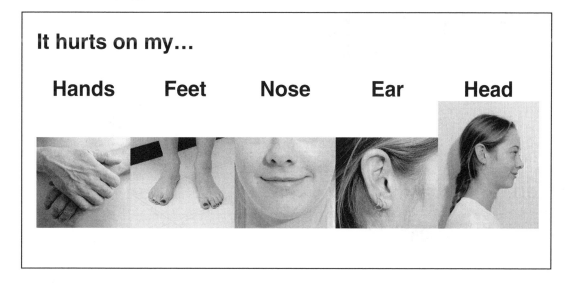

It hurts on my…

Hands     Feet     Nose     Ear     Head

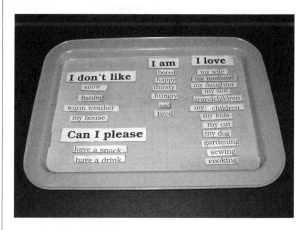

Message Magnets (Buettner, 1999)

## Pain assessments (*Continued*)

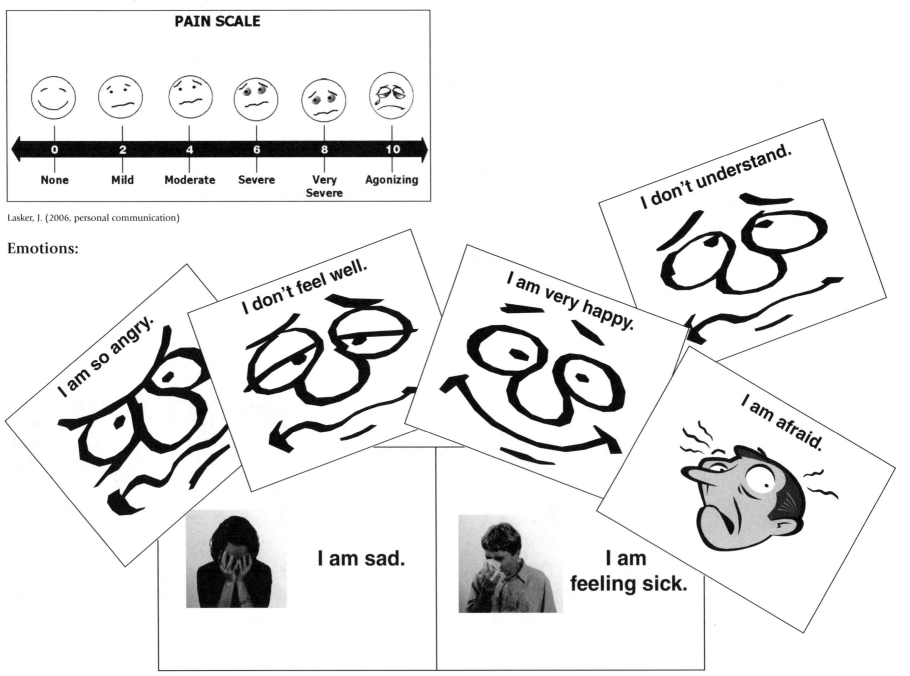

### PAIN SCALE

| 0 | 2 | 4 | 6 | 8 | 10 |
|---|---|---|---|---|---|
| None | Mild | Moderate | Severe | Very Severe | Agonizing |

Lasker, J. (2006, personal communication)

## Emotions:

I don't understand.

I don't feel well.

I am very happy.

I am so angry.

I am afraid.

I am sad.

I am feeling sick.

## Safety: The Prevention of Harm to Oneself or Others

At home:

**For HELP call**

# 9 1 1

**Turn off the stove.**

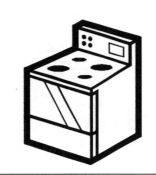

**Turn off the lights.**

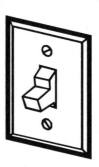

**I use my walker to be safe.**

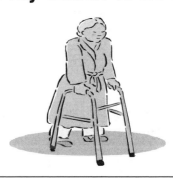

**Lock the door.**

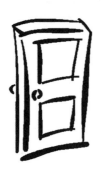

**Before I sit down in my wheelchair, I will:**

**1. Feel for the chair with my legs.**

**2. Reach back for the arm rests.**

**I use a wheelchair to get around.**

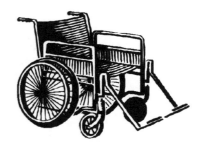

Medication safety:

Safety in the hospital:

## I take my pills after breakfast, at noon, and before bed.

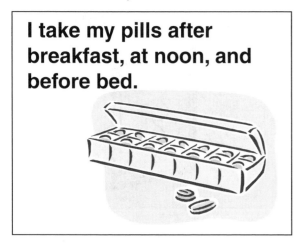

## I take my pills daily.

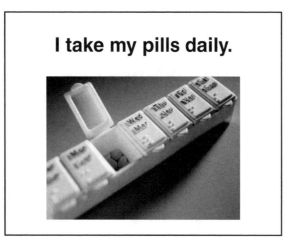

## Press the button to call the nurse.

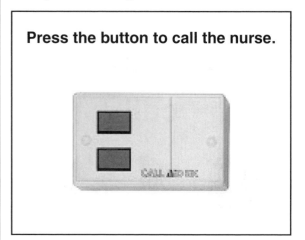

## I take my pills 3 times a day

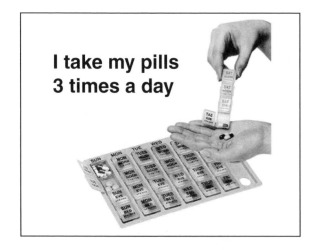

## I take my medicine to feel better.

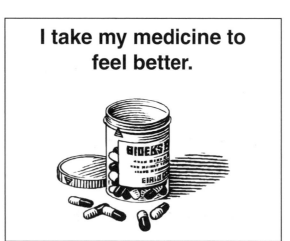

## I push the button for help.

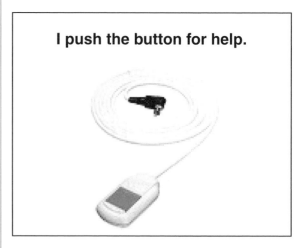

## Safety in the hospital (*Continued*)

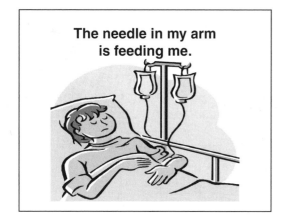

The needle in my arm is feeding me.

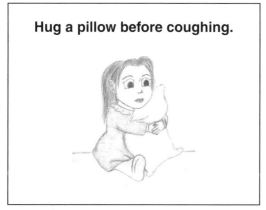

Hug a pillow before coughing.

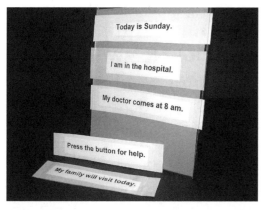

Today is Sunday.

I am in the hospital.

My doctor comes at 8 am.

Press the button for help.

My family will visit today.

## Tabletop Message Board: Hospital Safety Precautions

I broke my hip. I can't stand by myself.

I had heart surgery. I need help to stand up.

I hug a pillow when I laugh or cough.

I need to eat and drink what the nurse brings me.

I need help to go to the bathroom.

I will choke if I drink anything.

If I'm thirsty I can have ice chips.

I press this button to call the nurse.

This tube in my nose/stomach feeds me.

I am only allowed to drink clear liquids.

I will choke if I eat solid food.

These tubes in my arm help me get well.

The tube in my nose helps me breathe.

## Safe eating and feeding:

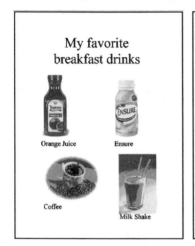

My favorite
breakfast drinks

Orange Juice    Ensure

Coffee

Milk Shake

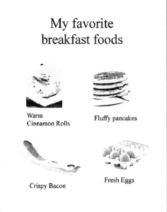

My favorite
breakfast foods

Warm
Cinnamon Rolls    Fluffy pancakes

Crispy Bacon    Fresh Eggs

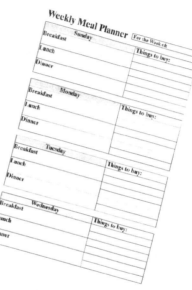

Weekly Meal Planner

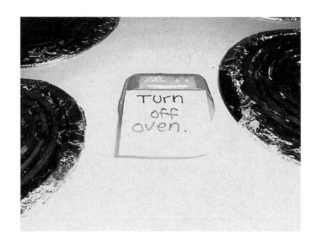

Turn off oven.

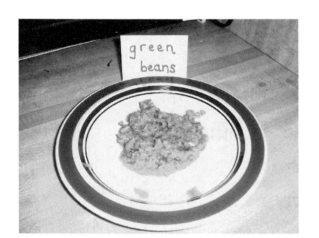

green beans

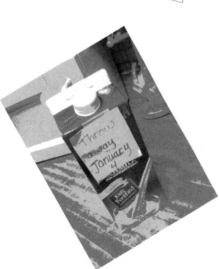

Throw away January 4

**Safe Swallowing Card**

1. **Take small bites, chew and swallow.**
2. **Take tiny sips.**
3. **Tuck your chin.**
4. **Double swallow after each sip.**

Personal hygiene:

| Using the Toilet: |
|---|
| Pull down my pants. |
| Sit down. |
| Do my business. |
| Wipe with paper. |
| Flush. |
| Pull up my pants. |
| Wash my hands. |

| Brushing my teeth: |
|---|
| Put water on the brush. |
| Put paste on the brush. |
| Brush all my teeth. |
| Spit. |
| Rinse. |
| Wipe my mouth. |
| Put away brush. |

| I use the toilet at: | |
|---|---|
| 7 a.m. | ✓ |
| 10 a.m. | ✓ |
| 1 p.m. | ✓ |
| 5 p.m. | |
| 9 p.m. | |

| Countdown to Laundry Day... | |
|---|---|
| ✓ | I changed my clothes. |
| ✓ | I changed my clothes. |
| | I changed my clothes. |
| | I changed my clothes. |
| | I changed my clothes. |
| | I changed my clothes. |
| | Laundry Day! |

| I eat at: | | |
|---|---|---|
| 7 a.m. | breakfast | ✓ |
| 10 a.m. | lunch | ✓ |
| 1 p.m. | tea time | ✓ |
| 5 p.m. | dinner | |
| 9 p.m. | warm milk | |
| | | |

## Personal hygiene (*Continued*)

**I trim my beard daily.**

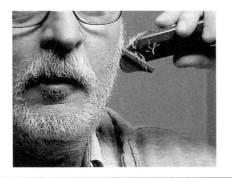

**I need to change my clothes every day.**

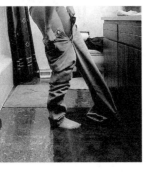

| **My Bathroom Schedule** | |
|---|---|
| | **Take a bath.** |
| | **Dry off.** |
| | **Button my shirt.** |
| | **Put on my pants.** |
| | **Put on my socks.** |
| | **Brush my teeth.** |
| | **Flush the toilet.** |

# CHAPTER 5

# Using Memory Aids to Increase Engagement and Activity

## Problems with Lack of Engagement or Activity

Many individuals with memory impairment seem to lose interest in their familiar hobbies or activities; they may appear apathetic or depressed about life. When questioned about what they might like to do, they cannot think of anything to suggest. When asked to do a specific activity or to go on an outing, they may decline the invitation. Before assuming the person is really not interested in doing anything, consider that the memory impairment might be the culprit. The person may not be able to remember the specific activities he or she would enjoy or cannot remember the words to describe them. The person may not recognize the words used to invite him or her to do something or may not understand them. Written and graphic memory supports can be very helpful for maintaining interest and engagement in preferred activities and hobbies. A visual prompt may be more effective than the verbal cue because objects and written words are permanent and static; in comparison, auditory information in the form of words, phrases, and sentences is transient, often disappearing into thin air before it is fully processed and understood.

Please note! While it may be the goal of family and professionals to increase engagement in activities by their person with memory impairment, the activities will need to be meaningful and desirable to the person for him or her to want to participate. Life-long hobbies and interests will always attract more attention and interest than generic recreational activities designed for the older adult. Buettner and Martin (1995) and Eisner (2001) have written guidebooks for the professional and family caregiver that focus on selecting and modifying activities that will allow the individual to engage meaningfully in his or her own preferred interests. When the individual's cognitive impairments prevent the enjoyment of an activity that requires complex skills, the author suggests ways to modify or simplify the activities such that they can continue to be enjoyed. For example, the formerly expert bridge player may not be able to participate in a competitive bridge match because of memory impairments, but would find other, simpler card games, like gin rummy, to be enjoyable. The former accountant may enjoy counting out and wrapping coins to deposit in the bank. The homemaker known for her delicious baked goods may feel more confident when using a large-print, illustrated cookbook or recipe cards to support her in the kitchen.

The following memory aids are designed to be used to support memory for complex activities (like using a cell phone or the TV remote control), to alert and trigger memory for familiar activities, and to engage the individual with interesting and comforting materials. There is increasing research evidence to support the notion that appropriate engagement in activities and with materials prevents disruptive or maladaptive behaviors from occurring. The person who is occupied with an interesting task or activity will be happier, and less likely to become upset or agitated, than the person who is left alone and without any means of stimula-

tion. Creative modifications to familiar activities have been shown to maintain interest in lifelong hobbies. For example, the former quilter may no longer be able to use a needle to sew but will still be interested in matching fabrics of different patterns and shapes. Similarly, the former professional musician may no longer be able to play the violin, but will be very interested in reading about famous composers or identifying different orchestral instruments from pictures or audiotapes.

## Examples of Memory Aids

In the early stages of memory impairment, it is the more complex familiar routines and information that begin to be problematic, such as learning to use a cell phone or to navigate home media with several different remote controls. The constant changing and upgrading of computers and computer software require learning and re-learning multiple steps and procedures for accessing familiar programs. Written lists of procedures are helpful at all stages of electronic use, from when first learning a new system, to later when a written list is a comforting support in the event that part of the procedure is forgotten. The following examples are generic instruction lists; each individual electronic device will have a unique

set of operating instructions that will need to be written down in a simple format. It may take a couple of tries to get a usable system; it is helpful to have one person describe all the actions being taken to operate the equipment, while a second person is writing down the steps. Review what was written, simplifying the language and eliminating redundant words, then follow the written instructions. You will know immediately if something has been left out or if there are extra unnecessary steps; revise accordingly.

## Written Instruction Cards

| To check e-mail on your computer: |
| --- |
| 1. Press [power] button |
| 2. Wait until icons appear at the bottom of screen. |
| 3. Using the mouse, move the arrow to the Outlook icon. |
| 4. Click the left mouse button. |
| 5. Read through the list of mail messages. |
| 6. Using the mouse, move the arrow to the message you want to read. |
| 7. Click the left mouse button. |
| 8. Read your message. |

**Written Instruction Cards** (*Continued*)

---

**Cell Phone:** Checking my messages

1. Press blue line to select **Menu**
2. Press > until **Messages** appears
3. Press blue line to select
4. Press blue line to listen
5. Listen to messages
6. Press 7 to **delete** message
7. Press blue line to **end**

---

**Cell Phone:** Calling a friend

1. Press blue line to select **Menu**
2. Press blue line to select
   **PhoneBook**
3. Press blue line to select **find**
4. Type first letter of friend's name
5. Press blue line to select OK
6. Press > until friend's name appears
7. Press blue line to **Call**
8. Talk to friend
9. Press **Stop** to end call

---

**Remote Controls:**
**To watch Cable TV**

1. Press [cable] button on Comcast
   remote
2. Press [power] button on Comcast
   remote
3. Press [TV] button on Sony remote
4. Press [power] button on Sony
   remote
5. To change channel, Press button
   on Sony remote
6. To change volume, Press [+] or [−]
   button on Sony remote

---

Other complex and commonly forgotten procedures include: how to operate the ATM machine, how to pump gas at a self-service station, and directions to familiar locations.

## Calendars and Planners

As memory lapses become more noticeable, keeping track of activities and appointments can become challenging and the fear of forgetting them can become stressful. The home calendar, either on the wall or by the telephone, is the most common and natural memory support that most people use. Calendars come in all sizes and varieties; the wipe-off style of wall calendar that has a magnetized back for affixing to the refrigerator is very popular. The usefulness of the calendar will depend on the legibility of the information written on it and the frequency with which it is consulted. Activities and appointments should be written clearly, with the time noted, and large enough to be read from a distance. If multiple family members' activities are written on the same calendar, it can be very useful to color-code the messages (red for Mom, blue for Dad, green for Brother, and yellow for Sister). The calendar should be placed in a location that is clearly visible to family members as soon as they enter the room; the more often the calendar is read, the more likely the relevant information on the calendar will be remembered. When memory problems become more apparent, it can be valuable to decide on routine times of the day to review the calendar. If the calendar is in the kitchen, it may not be too difficult to plan to look at it everyday while eating breakfast. Find today's date and read the appointments or activities planned. At the end of the day, or at dinner time, review the calendar again; check off the day and the activities accomplished; write any new plans on the appropriate day and move those that were not done today to another day.

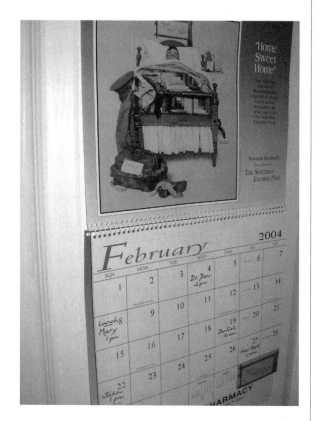

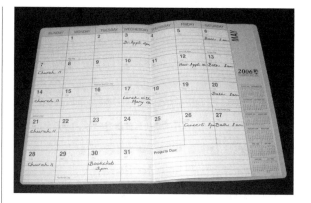

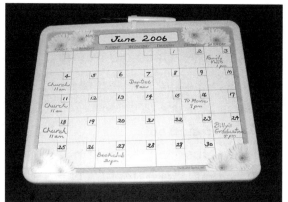

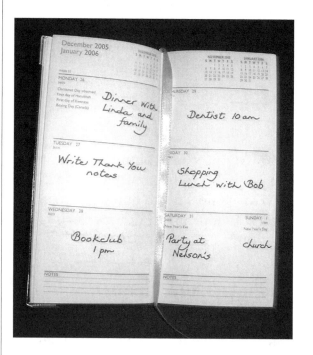

Portable calendars, in the form of planners, serve the same function of remembering activities and appointments when people are away from home. Similarly, planners come in many sizes and formats. Again, their usefulness is dependent on the legibility of the notes made and the frequency to which it is referred.

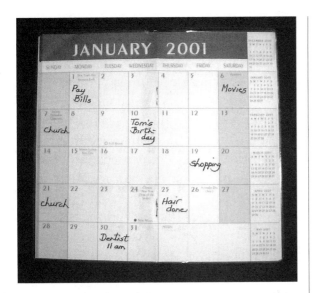

The benefits of routinely using a planner include: 1) the confidence of knowing the important information you need is at your fingertips, 2) new information can be written into the planner immediately and not forgotten, and 3) other information can be included in your planner, such as telephone directory, address book, and lists. For those individuals who are beginning to notice memory lapses for peoples' names and other common facts, it can be very helpful to include lists of words and names, in relevant categories, in the planner. For example, lists of names labeled, "Church friends," "Work friends," "Neighbors," and "Family" can be written down at a time when there is no pressure to remember them; then before going to church, for example, the "Church friends" list can be read quickly and those names refreshed. Easier name recall has been reported by those individuals who have tried this memory strategy.

**Church Friends**

**Bob and Mary Smith**
**Kay Ledgerville**
**Sharon and Ray Jones**
**Karen Howard**
**Pastor Jim Fellows**

**Things to Do**

**Dry cleaners**
**Go to vet**
**Call Dr. Barlow**
**Buy birthday gift for Jo**

**Shopping List**

**Milk**
**Dog food**
**Lettuce & cucumbers**
**Order birthday cake**
**Candles and napkins**

When memory interferes with remembering lifelong hobbies and interests, the following written and graphic supports can maintain familiar information and facilitate engagement in pleasurable activities.

**Remembering what you like to do:**

**Things I like to do in my spare time:**

Take a walk

Watch TV

Water the plants

Fold the laundry

Set the table

**Remembering what you like to do**
(*Continued*)

| My hobbies and interests: |
| --- |
| Gardening<br><br>Crocheting<br><br>Flower arranging<br><br>Singing in the choir<br><br>Aerobics<br><br>Traveling |

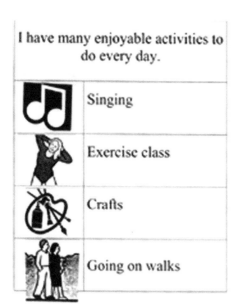

I have many enjoyable activities to do every day.

| | |
| --- | --- |
| ♫ | Singing |
| | Exercise class |
| | Crafts |
| | Going on walks |

## Reading as an Activity or Favorite Pastime

For the person who loves to read, there are two problems with the reading materials themselves that may explain loss of interest in reading. First, the size of the print or type may be too small to read easily. The solution to this problem is to find large-type reading materials; several popular monthly publications, such as *Reader's Digest*, are available in a larger font size. Similarly, most bookstores now carry a large-print section with a variety of books in the easier-to-read fonts.

Second, the complexity of the reading material may challenge memory capacity. That is, technical topics, literary, and abstract writing require a variety of cognitive resources to decode, understand, remember, and analyze the text. Most reading materials require that each sentence read be stored temporarily in short-term or working memory until the next sentence is read and processed in relation to the previous one. Persons with memory impairments may not have access to all of the cognitive resources needed to appreciate what they are reading, or to hold onto each successive sentence until the story or idea of the text is understood. They may find themselves reading and re-reading the same sentence or paragraph; this can become frustrating and less than pleasurable. Family may notice the person reading less frequently, or not at all. The solution to this is to provide reading materials that are less complex or technical, and to modify reading materials to enhance reading pleasure. For example, the scientist who spent his professional career reading technical journals may enjoy magazines for the lay public on science topics, such as *Discover, Popular Mechanics,* and *Psychology Today.* Readers of literary fiction may enjoy re-reading the classics of their youth (e.g., *Tom Sawyer, Anne of Green Gables, The Yearling*), more recent young adult fare (e.g., the *Harry Potter* series), or high-interest/low-vocabulary reading materials designed for younger students. Reading aloud children's literature or storybooks to grandchildren can remain pleasurable for some persons in the latter stages of dementia. Reading materials designed specifically for persons with dementia are beginning to be published (see Lydia Burdick's *The Sunshine on My Face,* Health Professions Press, 2005).

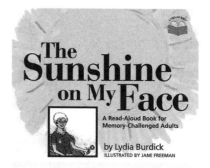

## Interest Albums

When reading becomes less pleasurable because of memory impairments, a good substitute for the book lover is the interest album. This collection of pictures with some large-print words about a single, favorite topic or activity can provide many hours of engagement. Interest albums can be made using magazine pictures, photographs of familiar and personal objects, and mementos and memorabilia that are often included in scrapbooks. The pictures below are just a sample of the infinite topics possible to depict in an interest album, such as baseball or other sports, a doll collection, wine, fishing, music, theatre, reading, TV shows, movies/actors, gardening, shopping, birds, favorite trips, and so forth.

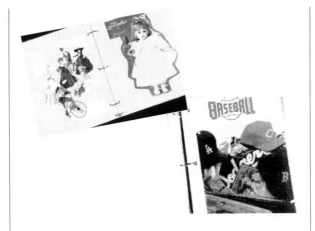

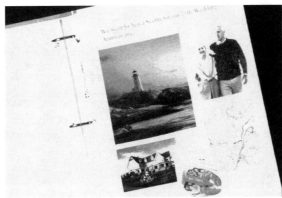

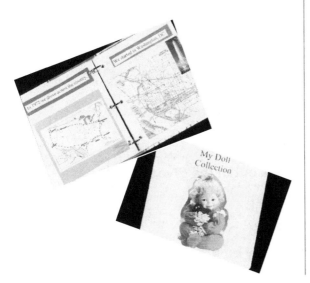

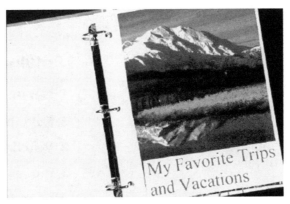

## Home Decorator Books

These nontext books (Buettner, 1999) were designed to substitute for women's decorating magazines when the print was too small and the information too complex for pleasure reading. Manipulation of the tactile materials, including fabric, wallpaper, paint, and carpet scraps, has been shown to elicit conversation on the topic of home decoration.

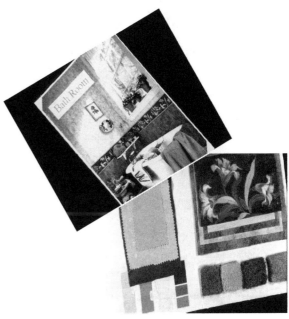

# Modifying Activities to Include Written Cues

## Religious Activities:

### Laminated Prayer Cards

> **The Lord is my Shepherd;**
>
> **I shall not want.**
>
> **He maketh me to lie down in green pastures.**
>
> **He leadeth me beside the still waters.**
>
> **He restoreth my soul.**

---

> **Shema** שמצ
>
> שמעישראל **Shema Yisrael,**
>
> ייאלהינו **Adonai Eloheinu**
>
> ייאהד **Adonai Echad!**
>
> ברוקשמכבוד **Baruch sheim kevod**
>
> מלכותלעולמומעד **Malchuot leolam vaed!**

## Message Magnets: Prayers and Old/New Testament Sort

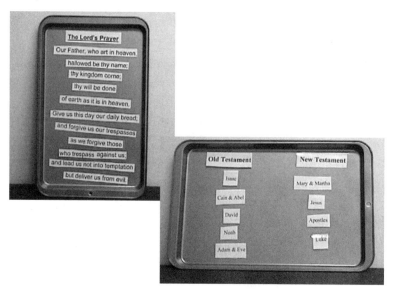

(Courtesy of Joanne Lasker, Ph.D., and Angela Halter, M.S., Florida State University. Reproduced with permission.)

## Around-the-House Activities:

### Laminated Activity Cards

> **Folding the Laundry**
>
> 1. **Get the clothes out of the dryer.**
> 2. **Fold the towels.**
> 3. **Match the socks.**
> 4. **Put clean laundry on dresser.**

## Wash the dishes

1. Fill the sink with warm water.
2. Wash the dish.
3. Rinse the dish.
4. Put the dish on rack.
5. Wash the next one.

## Feed the birds

1. Get the birdseed.
2. Open the cage and get food dish.
3. Pour birdseed into dish.
4. Place dish in cage.
5. Latch the cage door.

## Water the plants

1. Fill the watering can with water.
2. Water the plants in the kitchen.
3. Water the plants in the den.
4. Put the watering can away.

Cooking: Step-by-step instructions

## Making Coffee

1. Fill coffee carafe with water.
2. Pour water into coffee maker.
3. Measure coffee using spoon.
4. Put coffee into coffee filter.
5. Close filter door.
6. Press <ON> button.

## Making Lunch with Microwave

1. Get lunch dish out of fridge.
2. Put dish in microwave.
3. Close microwave door.
4. Press <2-0-0-Time>.
5. Wait for time to ring.
6. Remove dish and eat lunch.

A variety of illustrated cookbooks are available including, *Look 'n Cook Microwave: Easy-to-Make Illustrated Recipes* (Sudol, 1999), and *Home Cooking* (Attainment Company, Appendix D).

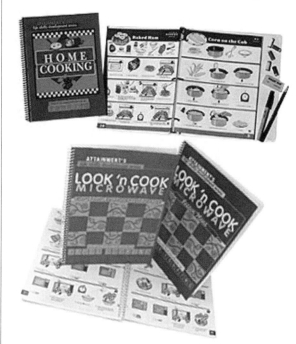

## Sorting Tasks: Stamps, Coupons, Cards

Coupons can first be cut from sales circular and then sorted by category (Montessori activity; Camp, 1999)

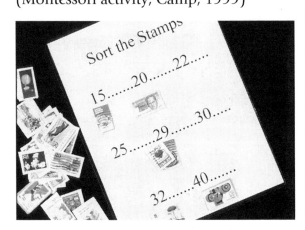

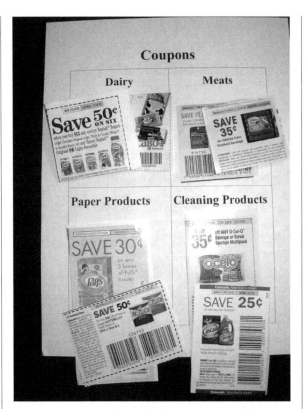

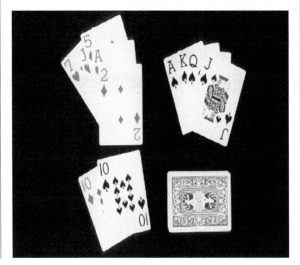

## Memory Boxes: Collections with a Theme without Written Cues for Tactile Manipulation

Sewing basket

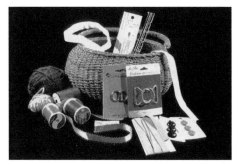

Travel souvenirs

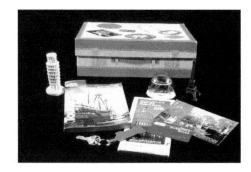

My purse

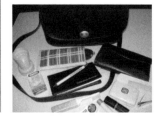

## Theme Boxes with Written Cues: Objects + Cue Cards (songs, stories)

### Christmas

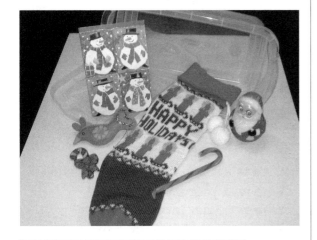

### White Christmas

I'm dreaming of a white Christmas
Just like the ones I used to know
Where the tree tops glisten
And children listen
To hear sleigh bells in the snow.

I'm dreaming of a white Christmas
With every Christmas card I write
May your days be merry and bright
And may all your Christmases be white.

### Home for the Holidays

Oh, there's no place like home for the holidays,
'Cause no matter how far away you roam,
When you pine for the sunshine of a friendly gaze,
For the holidays, you can't beat home, sweet home.

## Other Themes: School Days, Thanksgiving, Halloween, Easter, Passover, Shabbat

### Hanukkah

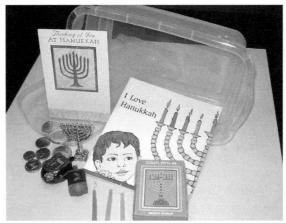

### Dreidel

Dreidel, dreidel, dreidel
I made it out of clay
And when it's dry and ready
Oh, dreidel I will play.

## Other Song Cards

### Kisses Sweeter than Wine

Well, when I was a young man never been kissed
I got to thinkin' it over how much I had missed
So I got me a girl and I kissed her and then, and then
Oh, lordy, well I kissed 'er again

Because she had kisses sweeter than wine
She had, mmm, mmm, kisses sweeter than wine.

### Mr. Tambourine Man

Hey, Mister Tambourine Man, play a song for me
I'm not sleepy and there ain't no place I'm goin' to
Hey, Mister Tambourine Man, play a song for me
In the jingle, jangle morning, I'll come followin' you

Take me for a trip upon your magic swirlin' ship
All my senses have been stripped
And my hands can't feel to grip
And my toes too numb to step
Wait only for my boot heels to be wanderin'

### Lemon Tree

When I was just a lad of ten, my father said to me
Come here and take a lesson from the lovely lemon tree
Don't put your faith in love, my boy, my father said to me
I fear you'll find that love is like the lovely lemon tree

Lemon tree, very pretty, and the lemon flower is sweet
But the fruit of the poor lemon is impossible to eat
Lemon tree, very pretty, and the lemon flower is sweet
But the fruit of the poor lemon is impossible to eat

## Group Activities

Group activities can be enhanced with written cue cards

### Current Affairs:

---

**Hurricanes**

I survived hurricane Kate in 2005.

The roof of my house blew off.

The Red Cross has a shelter in our local high school.

I moved to a safer house with my cat.

---

**The War in Iraq**

President Bush declared war on Iraq in 2003.

We support our young men and women in the service.

They are fighting to establish democracy in Iraq.

A new government was recently elected in Iraq.

---

### Discussion Topics:

---

**Advice on Marriage**

What is the secret to a good marriage?

What makes a good spouse?

Tips for getting along with the relatives.

Tips on raising the kids.

Issues of money and finances

---

**Planting a Garden**

What to plant?
When to start preparing the soil?
What type of fertilizer?
When do you weed?
When do you harvest?

---

**Solar Power**

What is it?
Will it save money?
Will it protect the environment?
What happens on a rainy day?
What about other sources of power, like windmills?

---

**Famous People in Sports**

What do you remember about:
Roger Bannister
Joe DiMaggio
Hank Aaron
Babe Ruth
Casey Stengel
Lou Gehrig
Mohammed Ali

---

**Favorite TV Shows**

Let's talk about our favorite TV shows:

Who was your favorite actor?
Who was your favorite actress?
What variety shows did you watch?
Which news programs did you like?

What do you remember about:
The Ed Sullivan Show
The Honeymooners
I Love Lucy
Lassie
Father Knows Best
Flipper

---

**Going on Vacation**

Where shall we go?
What should we pack?
How much money do we need?
Who should go with us?
Do we plan our own itinerary?
Or should we take a guided tour?
Do we need immunizations?
Do we need a passport?
How long should our trip be?

# CHAPTER 6

# Using Memory Aids to Modify Difficult Behaviors

The most common behavior challenges that have been addressed successfully with written memory supports include repetitive questions, expressions of anxiety and fear, and physical agitation. Many of the most difficult situations for caregivers to handle on a daily basis are the repetitive questions or statements made by their loved one. It is the rare person who can answer the same question repeatedly or explain away a worry, concern, or fear time after time without getting angry or frustrated themselves. One caregiving husband reported the usefulness of a particular page in his wife's memory book for helping her to remember her home. He reported that every evening after dinner she would thank him for the lovely meal, put on her coat, and then ask to be taken home. When this "sundowning" behavior first started, he would try to explain to her that she was at home, showing her familiar objects around the house. Sometimes the only way to comfort her was to go along with her misconception, get in the car, drive around the block, and then come "home." After dinner on one cold, snowy day when he did not want to risk their lives in the car, he decided to show her the page in her memory book that stated, "I have lived in this house at 123 Elm Street for 52 years." Surprisingly, she looked at the page and remarked, "Oh yes, that's right" and removed her coat. Her husband reported great satisfaction with using the memory book to prevent her sundowning behaviors.

A caregiving daughter expressed much frustration with her father's daily requests for her mother's whereabouts. She would patiently explain everyday that her mother (his wife) had died 3 years previously; he would express complete surprise and disbelief at the "news," and they would both end up crying. A memory book page that stated, "My wife, Lillian, died of liver cancer in 1995 and is resting peacefully in Woodlawn Gardens," with a photograph of her gravestone, prompted his response, "Oh, that's where she is." His daughter reported that she could hand him the memory book opened to that page whenever he would ask about his wife, but that he eventually stopped asking. He spent much of his time looking at his memory book, especially that page.

The persistent, daily aggravations that caregivers experience because of the inability of their loved one to remember the answer to the question they just asked or the explanation of the concern they just expressed can be addressed by making a written reminder or response to the question or concern. These reminders can be in the form of a memory book page, as the examples above illustrate, or they can be written down in a format that seems logical and practical to the situation, including fake letters, memo boards, and reminder cards. The following are examples of a variety of written reminder formats for representative repetitive behaviors.

**One important note!** Sometimes caregivers think the person might be asking questions repeatedly just to get attention or to aggravate them. A simple way to determine whether the repetitive question is being asked to gain attention from the caregiver or to seek information that has been forgotten is to ask the person his or her own question. If he or she knows the answer, the purpose of the questioning is to seek attention; figure out some ways to engage this person in a meaningful activity and, if possible,

direct him or her to another activity with other people. If the person does not know the answer to the question, then he or she needs a written memory support.

## Reducing Repetitive Questions and Behaviors

1. Memory Book Page
   When there is a page in the memory book that answers the repetitive question, caregivers can refer the person to that page when the question arises.

   > "I think the answer to that question is in your book; here, read this."

   > "I believe I read something about that in this book; what does it say here?"

---

**I have lived at 321 Elm Street for 52 years.**

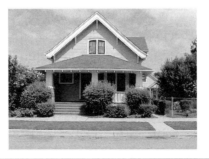

---

**My wife Jane lost her valiant fight with cancer on May 10, 1999 and rests peacefully here.**

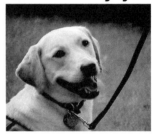

---

**Buster was my favorite dog. He was my best friend for many years.**

---

2. Fake/Proxy/Pseudo Letter
   **Problem:** Person is worried that he has not paid his income taxes or received his monthly pension check that is actually directly deposited in the bank. Caregiver repeatedly reminds him that he paid the taxes or the check is in the bank.

**Solution:** Create a proxy or pseudo letter from the IRS or the bank by photocopying a letter from the IRS or bank received in the past; cut and paste the official identifying information onto a blank paper; type a new, reassuring letter; and make multiple copies for future use. When the person asks about his tax or banking situation, the caregiver can respond, "Here is a letter you just received about that, what does it say?" Caregivers report that persons will then tell them the relevant information, and keep the paper to reread periodically until they forget about that concern.

---

**Parkvale**
SAVINGS BANK

February 28, 1996

Mr. John Doe
1234 Main Street
Anytown, USA 12345

Dear Mr. Doe,

　　As one of our Direct Deposit Customers, we would like to confirm that your Social Security and Pension checks have been arriving on time and are being depositied directly into your savings account on the first day of every month. If there were ever to be a problem, we would contact you immediately.

Thank you for your business. We value you as a customer in good standing.

Sincerely,


Jane Smith
Customer Service Representative
Suburban Branch

---

Internal Revenue Service
Washington, DC  20050

June 12, 2004

Mr. John  Doe
1234 Main Street
Anytown, USA 12345

Dear Mr. Doe,

　　We have received your income tax return for the year 2003.  Your tax refund was directly deposited into your savings account at Parkvale Savings Bank.

Thank you.

Jane Smith
Tax Accounting Specialist

---

3. Memo Board

**Problem:** Person is physically active, paces or walks around the house, giving the impression that she is looking for something, or is not sure where she is going. Caregiver complains that the pacing is troublesome and sometimes becomes accelerated, frantic, or agitated. Caregiver's efforts to redirect the person to a different activity or to stop the pacing are met with resistance or are ignored.

**Solution:** Create a memory area using a wipe-off memo board and/or magnetic or cork board. The refrigerator is often a good place to put this board; alternatively, the best place for a memo board is on the wall at eye level along the pacing path. It needs to be in a location that is passed frequently along the person's pacing route so that there are many opportunities to see it.

Write simple messages in large, clear printed letters on the board. These messages should address the person's concerns and the caregiver's suggestions for desirable alternate activities. For example, one person repeatedly asked what day it was and walked around the house looking for things to do. Her caregiver wrote the day's date ("Today is . . .") and a couple of reasonable activities (fold the laundry, water the plants). When she continued walking, she encountered the laundry basket in one room, the watering can in another, and she would stop to complete those activities.

Another person became worried about her husband when he left her home alone to do an errand; she would look for him all around the house and then would call her children, friends, and neighbors looking for him. The caregiver was advised to make a memo board and write on it, "John is at Lowe's. Will be home at 3 o'clock." It was assumed that she read the board repeatedly because she stopped telephoning others to find him.

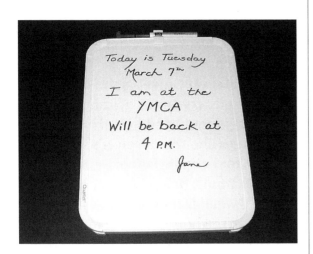

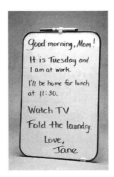

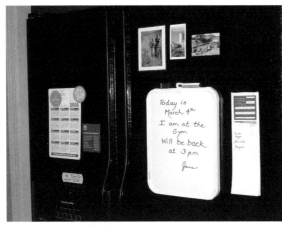

4. Reminder Cards
   Some caregivers report that the repeated questions or concerns are sometimes unpredictable in content and sometime recur on a random basis, from day to day or from one week to another. Sometimes the repeated questions or concerns occur in public places and create uncomfortable situations for the caregiver. A

lightweight, easy-to-carry system for writing down the answer to the question or concern is the solution to this problem. Index cards, or small memo notebooks, are easily kept in a purse, in the car, or in a coat pocket with a pen or pencil. When a question or concern arises, the answer can be written down and the card or notebook handed to the person to be read, and re-read as needed.

**Problem:** Caregiver and person are driving in the car to the grocery store. Person asks, "So, where are we going?" Caregiver responds, "We're going to the grocery store." Person nods, looks out the window, and 2 minutes later repeats the question.

**Solution:** This caregiver can make a reminder card that says "We're going to the grocery store" when stopped at the next red light. She can hand it to the person and say, "Here, read this."

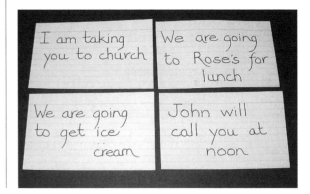

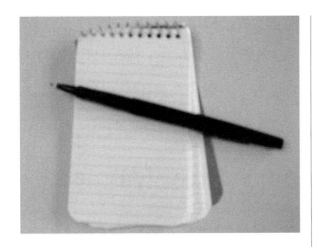

Another caregiver's spouse kept asking him what they were going to do that day. The caregiver made a card that listed several times and activities such as:

---

**Today's Events**

**9:00 Watch TV**
**Noon Eat lunch**
**2:00 Grocery store**
**5:00 Eat dinner**

---

**Honey-do List**

**Wash the dishes.**
**Empty the trash.**
**Sweep the porch.**

**I love you! ♥**

---

## Reducing Problems in the Nursing Home

Reminder cards can be useful to professional caregivers as well. **Nursing assistants** can carry a pen and some cards in their pocket and write a reminder message whenever and wherever they encounter a

---

*My daughter will visit me on Saturday.*

---

*My son called me last night.*

---

*My money is safe in the bank.*

---

person who is confused, fearful, agitated, or has a pressing concern.

A useful instructional handout, "Reminder Cards: Using Written Cues in the Home and Nursing Home," is included as Appendix B3. It can be helpful to keep a box with generic reminder cards at the nursing station for use whenever a concern arises.

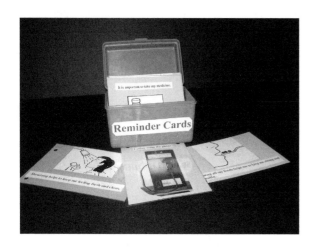

I live at

Magnolia

Nursing Home.

**Music activities**

**are free.**

**Meal Ticket**

_____ **Monday**

_____ **Tuesday**

_____ **Wednesday**

_____ **Thursday**

_____ **Friday**

_____ **Saturday**

_____ **Sunday**

The bathroom is

next to my room.

**Lunch is**

**served at noon**

**in the dining room.**

| Movie Pass | Movie Pass |
|---|---|
| | |

**Good for 1**
**FREE**
**Movie**

| Movie Pass | Movie Pass |
|---|---|

## Reducing Problems in Rehabilitation

Physical therapists (PTs) can use written reminder cards for a variety of repetitive tasks that persons with memory impairment need repeated reminders to accomplish. For example, safe ambulation, safe transfer, or use of a walker involves multiple steps that the PT often repeats verbally.

Instead, these steps can be written on a card and shown to the person during the task or taped within visual range for the person to see while he or she is completing the task.

Occupational therapists (OTs) can use reminder cards with or without illustrations to depict the multiple steps in various activities of daily living, such as dressing or grooming.

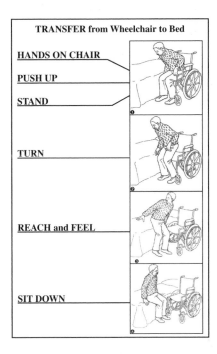

TRANSFER from Wheelchair to Bed

HANDS ON CHAIR

PUSH UP

STAND

TURN

REACH and FEEL

SIT DOWN

## Safe Walking

**Hold onto the walker.**
**Lift my foot.**
**Put it down.**
**Lift my other foot.**
**Put it down.**
**Lift the walker.**
**Move it forward.**
**Start over.**

## Standing Up from a Chair

**Hands on chair arms.**
**Knees together over toes.**
**Lean forward.**
**Push down on chair arms.**
**Lift off the chair.**

## Safe Transfer Steps

**Feet together straight ahead.**
**Knees over toes.**
**Lean forward.**
**Start to stand.**
**Swing hips to seat.**
**Move hand beyond seat.**
**Pivot and sit.**

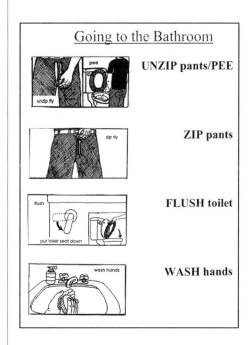

Going to the Bathroom

UNZIP pants/PEE

ZIP pants

FLUSH toilet

WASH hands

## To Shave

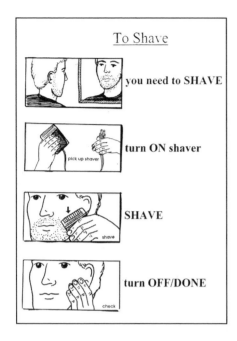

you need to SHAVE

turn ON shaver

SHAVE

turn OFF/DONE

## GET DRESSED

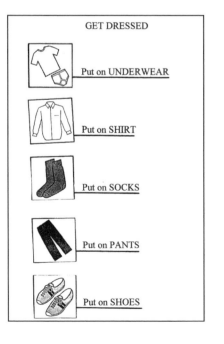

Put on UNDERWEAR

Put on SHIRT

Put on SOCKS

Put on PANTS

Put on SHOES

Speech-language pathologists (SLPs) can use written reminder cards for safe swallowing during meals, or for the multiple instructions in a swallowing evaluation.

---

## Safe Eating

Take a bite.
Chew and chew.
Swallow,
Take a sip.
Start over.

---

## Swallowing Evaluation

Take a sip/bite.
Keep it on my tongue.
Wait.
Swallow.

---

## More Examples of Written Supports

### Repetitive Questions

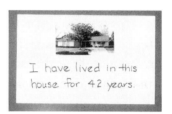

I have lived in this house for 42 years.

---

Max and I were great friends. I miss him since he died on March 13, 2005.

---

## Visitors' Log Book

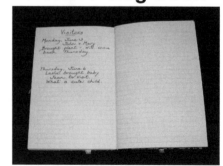

## Fears and Anxieties

I am safe here.

The Lord is watching over me.

My bill has been paid.

## Agitation Behaviors: Pacing, Repetitive Physical Behaviors

### *Tidy Bathroom Checklist*

_____ toilet paper
_____ soap
_____ paper towels

### *Energy Conservation*

**Turn off lights in:**

_____ bathroom
_____ bedroom
_____ kitchen
_____ den

*My job: Mail delivery*

**Get letters.
Read name.
Find person named.
Deliver their mail.**

*My job: Nametag check*

**Get nametags.
Read name.
Find person named.
Put nametag on.**

*My job: Set the table*

**Plate
Napkin
Fork-knife-spoon
Glass**

## Agitation Behaviors: Pacing, Repetitive Physical Behaviors (*Continued*)

---

*My job: Feed the birds*

**Get bird food.**
**Open cage.**
**Get food dish.**
**Pour food in dish.**
**Put dish in cage.**
**Close cage door.**

---

*My job: Watering plants*

_____ **kitchen**
_____ **bedroom**
_____ **den**

---

*My jobs:*

**Dust.**
**Fold the laundry.**
**Iron the clothes.**
**Sweep the kitchen.**

---

### Making the Salad

I need: **Bowl   knife   salad tongs**
　　　**Vegetables:** lettuce  tomatoes  carrots
　　　　　　　　　　radish  cucumbers  celery

**Chop the vegetables.**

**Tear the lettuce.**

**Put lettuce in bowl.**

**Put vegetables in bowl.**

**Toss the salad with tongs.**

---

### Washing the Clothes

**Make two piles: Darks and Lights**

Put dark clothes in washer.
Pour in 1 measure of detergent.
Start washer.
When done, put clothes in dryer.
When done, fold clothes.
Put folded clothes in basket.

Put light clothes in washer.
Pour in 1 measure of detergent.
Start washer.
When done, put clothes in dryer.
When done, fold clothes.
Put folded clothes in basket.

**Laundry is done!**

# CHAPTER 7

# Using Memory Aids in Adult Day Program, Assisted Living, and Nursing Home Settings

I n many residential and adult day program environments, the occupational therapist and the recreation therapist assume responsibility for finding ways to engage clients in meaningful communicative situations and activities. These therapists develop activity programs and related materials geared to the individual client's needs and abilities. Often these therapists come to learn the most about individual clients through scheduled conversation, current events, and reminiscence groups. They may be the most logical candidates for constructing memory wallets, memory books, and other written cuing systems, and for encouraging their use in daily recreational activities.

Volunteers, the mainstay of most therapeutic activity programs, are also excellent memory aid makers. Many program directors actively search for specific tasks in which to engage their volunteer staff because these individuals want to contribute positively to the well-being of the participants but are often at a loss for knowing what to do. Volunteers have enjoyed making memory books and memory wallets in adult day and nursing home settings. Because they spend many hours talking with clients, and often meet the families, they have commented that they have learned a great deal about the individuals from making the aids. For example, they usually have to verify factual information and obtain photographs from the family, who corrects confusions and provides additional factual information about the person's family and life. The Memory Aid Information Form for Nursing Homes (Appendix C2) can also be used to gather pertinent information.

## Memory Aids Facilitate Care Activities

In the nursing home or assisted living facility, it is the certified nursing assistant (CNA), however, who spends the most time with residents and is responsible for their daily care.

Their primary job is to make sure residents get up in the morning; get bathed, toileted, dressed, and groomed; eat their meals; take their medications; and get to bed at night. Their close, personal interactions with residents make them the most knowledgeable about resident likes and dislikes, individual patterns of behavior, and problem areas. As a result, they also have the most trouble with residents who do not understand their instructions, and who are uncooperative, agitated, or combative as a result of a memory-impairing illness. Nursing assistants, therefore, may be particularly receptive to interventions that improve communication between themselves and their residents.

Memory aids and written cuing systems have been particularly effective when CNAs have been consulted about their needs and specific tools are designed to address those concerns. For example, CNAs had been reported to be less than eager to implement memory book interventions to improve conversations with residents with dementia (Bourgeois, et al., 2001); they did not feel they had adequate time to stop their specific care duties to have a lengthy conversation with a resident using a memory book. Further, most communicative breakdowns occurred during the routine tasks of getting bathed, dressed, and fed, and

these activities were felt to take precedence over casual conversation. Therefore, as reported in Bourgeois et al. (2001), the memory book technology was modified in two ways to address these concerns: 1) memory books were reduced in size, weight, and content so that they could be carried with the residents to their activities; and 2) pages were included in their books that addressed the specific caregiving concerns of the CNAs. For example, if the resident was typically uncooperative about showering, a page that described showering in positive terms was included in the memory book.

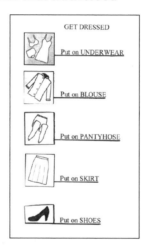

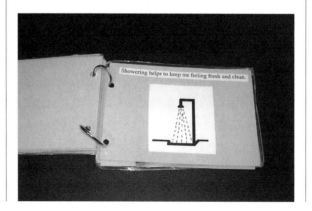

Nursing assistants were trained to use the memory books to increase cooperation during care activities; they were instructed to:

- Approach the resident from the front, gain eye contact, and smile.
- Greet the resident by name: "Good morning, Mrs. Smith."
- Introduce themselves and the activity: "I'm Anita and I'm here to help you get ready for the day."
- Show the memory book page for the activity: "Look at this, Mrs. Smith."
- Then guide the resident to the activity: "That says it's time for your shower now, so let's get up and get into that nice, warm shower."

As reported in Bourgeois et al. (2001, 2004), CNAs easily learned this positive communication routine and used the memory books to increase the cooperation of their residents. Nursing assistants noticed the value of using written cues to increase understanding and to decrease confusion; they were receptive to finding ways to ensure that the memory books were with residents throughout the day. This led to the creation of wearable devices (Appendix A) that allowed the memory book to be attached to the resident or to the person's clothing or wheelchair. A variety of lanyards, vests, aprons, and wheelchair bags were developed to accommodate the mobility needs of individual residents. Nursing assistants readily incorporated the attachment of the memory aid to the resident as part of their care routine; just as glasses and hearing aids were necessary for personal care completion, so too was the securing of the memory aid to the resident. Detailed instructions and patterns for making these wearable devices are included as Appendix A.

Because CNAs saw the value of written cues for their residents in the research study, they requested written cues for their other residents. This led to the

**Necklace**

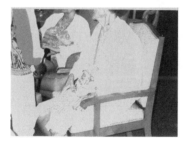

**Vest pocket**

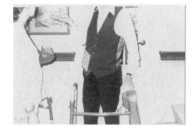

**Clip**

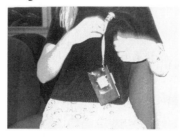

**Walker bag**

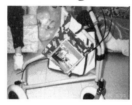

development of a collection of generic index cue cards that addressed a variety of care activity needs and other recurring repetitive questions that might arise with any resident on the unit. These cards were contained in an index box that was kept at the nurses' station and was available to anyone who needed a written cue card to allay a resident's concern. In addition, blank cards and a felt-tipped black ink pen were included in the box for staff members to write their own cue cards to address a unique concern of a resident. Bourgeois and Irvine (1999) have since created an interactive CD-ROM training program for CNAs that instructs them in

the procedures for creating effective reminder cards. A Reminder Card training handout is included in Appendix B3. These same instructions can be used to instruct family caregivers in the use of reminder cards for the unique repetitive question or concern that arises at unscheduled times, such as in the car on the way to an outing (i.e., church, the store, a doctor's appointment).

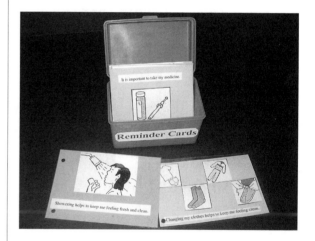

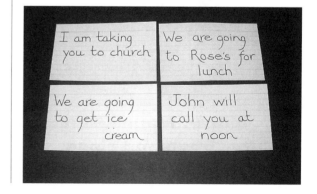

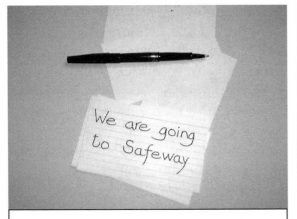

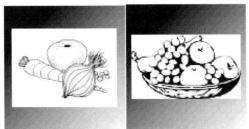

**Eating keeps me strong and healthy.**

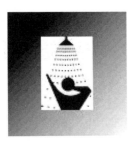

**Showering makes me feel fresh and clean.**

## Memory Aids Facilitate Activity Programs

Memory aids have been observed to facilitate many activities that become frustrating to both client and staff because of the individual's memory limitations. Specifically, group conversation or discussion activities are greatly enhanced when participants have a memory wallet or book to refer to; participants are observed to initiate statements, questions, and responses when they can prompt themselves with their memory aid. All individuals with memory aids can participate in group activities that may have been dominated by one or a few verbal participants in the past.

**When working with clients in a group:**

- Use memory aids to facilitate group discussions about families, life, jobs, and so forth.
- Choose one topic and ask all clients to talk about and show their wallet items on that topic, encouraging comments and questions among clients. For example, "Let's talk about what we did for a living. Show us the page about your profession."

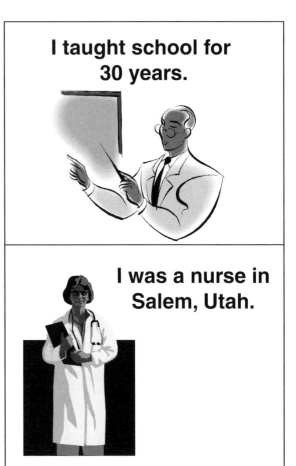

- Make up individualized Discussion Cards on conversational, current event topics prior to the activity. For example, if the topic is an upcoming presidential election, make up a list of five facts about elections and voting that each person would be able to state, call the family to verify the facts, and then write them down on a card for each person. The card might say:

### *Politics and Elections*

**I am a registered democrat.**

**I voted for Jimmy Carter in the last election.**

**My polling booth is at the Robinson Elementary School in Shaler.**

**I never ran for an elected post.**

**My nephew, John Smith, was elected mayor of Smithville in 1974.**

Another person's card would have five similar but personalized facts to use during the discussion.
- Add cards for field trips and other activities and then utilize for facilitating group discussion.

## MUSIC

**I enjoy all kinds of music.**

**I used to play the organ at my church.**

**Tommy Dorsey's Orchestra was one of my favorites.**

**I gave piano lessons to the neighborhood children years ago.**

**We had a player piano when I was a child.**

**I remember my father singing "I'm Looking Over a Four-Leaf Clover" while my sister and I pumped the pedals.**

### Janet, Beth, and I went to the zoo today.

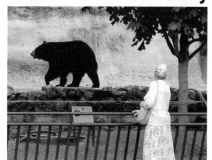

## Memory Aids Encourage Social Interaction

Social interaction between clients is also enhanced using memory aids. Individuals have been observed to initiate conversations with others by inviting them to look at their family pictures in their memory book. Nursing staff members have welcomed the change in residents' restlessness, constant complaining, and demands for attention when they can redirect these difficult behaviors using the memory aid as a catalyst for friendly conversations between clients.

Encourage your staff members and volunteers to use the wallets and memory books with the clients in the following ways:

1. **When talking with client alone:**

   - Ask the person to show you the wallet and to tell you about the items in it.
   - Talk about specific people when you're looking at the picture.
   - Assist individuals by reading along or prompting them to read the memory aid. For example, if a person has difficulty reading her statements, she may need a partner to "finger guide" her by pointing to her statements word by word as she reads them. This may help her to concentrate on the specific page and to tell you more about it.
   - Ask family members to make new pages with pictures and sentences to add to the wallet; or ask family members to send pictures for making new

---

**My grandson, Mark, graduated from Central Catholic High School on May 14, 2006.**

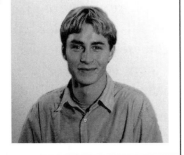

---

pages and then help the client make the pages (with picture and sentence) as new events occur, and add these to the wallet.

2. **When a client asks questions repeatedly:**

   - Make a page that states positively a fact related to the complaint.
   - Client complaint—"I am scared here."

   > *I am very safe here.*

3. **When a client asks the same question or makes a specific complaint:**

   - Have the person take out the wallet, help to find the correct page, and ask the person to read that to you OR
   - Make a reminder card with a positive statement that answers the concern and ask the person to read the card aloud.

   Getting clients to make positive verbal statements about a problem seems to redirect their thoughts/statements to positive ideas which you can reinforce by saying more about them.

   > *The staff takes good care of me.*

4. **When the client gets restless or engages in some activity that is nonproductive:**

   - Have the person get out the wallet and suggest that he or she use it to talk with a friend.

   There are many other possible uses of memory aids in adult day, assisted living, and nursing home settings. It will be important for professionals using these procedures, along with their own creative variations, to share these ideas and relevant data collected at professional conferences and in professional journals.

   > *I have many friends to talk to.*

# CHAPTER 8

# Using Memory Aids in the Home Environment with Family Members

## Helping Family Members Make and Use Memory Aids

The frustrations encountered by family members when a loved one has memory impairment can accumulate over time and create negative interactions. Spouses, other family members, children, and grandchildren may argue with, or attempt to quiz, the person to help him or her remember information pertinent to a particular situation. Repeated corrections lead to angry outbursts which often lead to avoidance—avoiding interactions with the person altogether. This unfortunate situation can be reversed by recruiting family members to be partners in the therapeutic process. Their primary role is to serve as the source of historical and current information about the person. They can provide the facts and information that will be most important to include in memory aids of all sorts. Because they experience the day-to-day frustrations of living with someone who has memory problems, they can describe the entire range of difficulties encountered in daily life. It is therefore critical to interview the family to find out specific frustrations and concerns, the difficult situations that arise on a regular basis, and what the members feel are the most pressing issues. The **Memory Aid Information form,** included as Appendix C1, is to be used to gather the relevant information about memory-related problems that can possibly be addressed with memory aids. In addition to biographical information that can be useful in developing a memory book or wallet, specific difficult or repetitive behaviors are solicited, as well as information about likes and dislikes, hobbies and interests, and the person's daily routine. Family members will also be important therapy partners in implementing and using the memory aids for the concerns they have expressed. They may help make the memory aids and then learn how to use them to reduce the frustrations that result from the memory impairment. Caregivers who have made memory books often report that they feel they are doing something concrete to help their family member; they enjoy the task of looking for old pictures and remembering happy occasions from the past, and the completed memory book is an attractive, interesting, and useful product for which they receive many compliments. Bourgeois (1997) has published a fill-in-the-blank memory book with tear-out instructions for family caregivers. Using memory aids, including memory books and reminder cards, to reduce the frequency of memory problems improves the interactions between family members and helps them feel more in control and competent in difficult situations. Caregiving spouses in a support group have been observed sharing their successes at reducing repetitive questions with a written reminder card; others facilitate workshops at support groups, nursing homes, and adult day centers to assist other families in developing memory books and interest albums.

The form, **Family Caregiver Instructions** (Appendix B1), was designed for family members who want to make memory aids. You, the professional, may need to review the instructions with the family members, emphasizing relevant points. Some family members will be quick to understand the procedures and will, in short course, return with a beautifully completed memory aid. Others, however, will need the process to be broken down into more manageable steps. These family members usually benefit from being assigned two preliminary tasks: 1) completing the Memory Aid Information Form (Appendix C1), and 2) finding relevant family pictures. At a subsequent visit, the professional can assist the family member with writing out, in short declarative sentences, the person's biography, daily schedule, family tree, and so forth. Selections from this written list can then be made, based on their importance to the person and the availability of pictures to accompany the sentences. Finally, pictures are matched to sentences and the actual assembly of the memory aid can begin.

In addition to the biographical, family, and daily schedule information, it is also helpful to ask family members to list recurrent questions that the person asks and other difficult behaviors that the person exhibits in order to develop pages, or other memory aids, that address those specific concerns. For instance, a woman whose father repeatedly asked the whereabouts of his deceased brother made a memory wallet page that included a picture of the brother's gravesite and the sentence, "My brother Tom died at the Battle of the Bulge on December 30, 1944." The woman gave her father the memory wallet and opened it to that page whenever he asked that question; she reported that her father stopped asking that question after about a week of having the memory aid.

Once the memory aid has been made, the **Guidelines for Having a Satisfying Conversation** (Appendix B2) is another useful handout to share with family members in order to help them feel more comfortable using the memory aid during conversations. Family members may need specific instructions for making and using reminder cards, or other visual cuing systems, such as planners, calendars, and memory boards. These instructions have been included on the handout, **Reminder Cards: Using Written Cues in the Home and Nursing Home,** included as Appendix B3.

## Using Memory Aids with Children

Children are often upset and confused by the forgetfulness of elderly relatives and friends who have memory-impairing illnesses, including Alzheimer's disease (AD). Explanations about the disease, its causes and course, may allay children's fears that they were somehow to blame for Grandpa's mean words, quick temper, or unresponsiveness. Yet, it may be difficult to encourage them to interact with their relative in positive ways after a particularly upsetting episode.

The following instructions provide a constructive, child-directed activity for children and their memory-impaired relative to complete together. Appendix B4 contains a reproducible **Memory Booklet** that children can use for making a memory aid with their memory-impaired relative or friend. Using the completed memory booklet provides a structured way for children to talk with the person. The format and text of the booklet ensures the maximum opportunity for the memory-impaired individual to succeed in the interaction. The use of large-print, simple sentences, one idea per page, and the sentence completion format takes advantage of the memory-impaired person's remaining reading skills; research has shown that these features successfully prompt accurate recall of factual information that is often confused by the person.

It is helpful to introduce the idea of memory impairment and its effects on communication and daily living with an educational session that involves reading a book about memory impairment with the child. The book *Grandpa Doesn't Know It's Me* (Guthrie, 1986) is an excellent choice to share with the young child in anticipation of discussing his or her own feelings, fears, and experiences with a memory-impaired relative. An annotated bibliography of other relevant books, with age appropriateness indicated, is included at the end of this chapter.

Once you feel the child has some understanding of the problems associated with memory impairment, and that he or she is not to blame for them, you are urged to explore with the child ways that he or she can interact positively with the person. The memory booklet is presented as one way to facilitate meaningful conversation between the child and the memory-impaired relative.

## How to Assist Children in Making Memory Aids

1. Set aside a period of time when you can be assured of minimal interruptions.
2. Explain to the child that you want to discuss the problems the family is experiencing with the memory-impaired relative. Ask the child to help you identify the various incidents that he or she has observed that indicate to him or her that the relative has changed. Ask the child to share with you how that makes him or her feel about the relative.
3. Explain the person's memory disorder, using terminology appropriate to the child's level of comprehension. Reading together one of the referenced books at the end of this booklet is an excellent way to share information about AD or other dementias.
4. Reassure the child that he or she is in no way responsible for the relative's problem behaviors and that any negative/aggressive behaviors toward the child or other family members are related to the disease and are not intentional.
5. Ask the child to tell you activities that he or she used to enjoy doing with the relative. Discuss why the relative may no longer be able to participate in those activities as he or she used to.
6. Ask the child to help you figure out things that he or she could do together with the relative that would be enjoyable and helpful. Write these down for future reference; before visiting the relative, have the child pick one or two of the activities to do with the relative during the visit. Be sure to review with the child what he or she intends to do and then later ask him or her to tell you about the outcome.

7. Suggest to your child that because the relative is forgetting so many important facts it would be helpful, and fun, to make a Book of Memories for him or her that they could talk about together.

8. Read the booklet with the child, pointing out that once completed the relative will be able to read the sentences and look at the pictures to remind him or her of people and events that he or she is having trouble remembering.

9. Gather supplies that the child will need to use for this activity, including scissors, glue stick, pencil with eraser, crayons, a 3-ring folder or binder, and photographs.

10. Assist the child in reviewing family photo albums for photographs to paste onto the appropriate pages. It is best to find pictures that show only one person; if necessary, photos that show two or more people should be clearly labeled with their names. If photos are unavailable, encourage the child to draw a picture depicting the person or idea in the space provided.

11. Once appropriate pictures are collected, explain to the child that he or she can show the booklet to the relative and say, "Grandpa, I would like us to make a book about your memories so that we can talk about them. I have pictures of all of our family and about your life to paste in the book. Will you help me to fill in the sentences so we can read it together later? You tell me how to finish these sentences and I'll write the words in for you."

12. Be prepared to monitor the activity initially. You may need to suggest that the child and the relative only complete one page, or two, per session. Encourage the child to end the activity by saying, "Thanks so much, Grandpa, for helping me to make this memory book. Let's do some more of it tomorrow." The relative may not want to part with the booklet; suggest to the child that he or she can let Grandpa look at the book until he is distracted by another activity and puts it down voluntarily. Then the child can retrieve it and put it in a safe place until the next session.

13. Once the booklet is completed, the child can tell the relative, "Grandpa, this book tells us all about you, your life, and your family. You can look at it whenever you want to remember these happy memories. Let's look at it together now. Please tell me all about these pictures."

14. Instruct the child to listen patiently to what the relative has to say about each picture. The relative may say the same things about the pictures each time they talk about them; reassure the child that this is good practice for the relative. The child can feel like he or she is helping the relative to rehearse the information that is difficult to remember.

15. Have the child point out details in the picture. For example, when the child and the relative are looking at the grandparents' wedding picture, the child could say, "look at the beautiful wedding dress Grandma was wearing" or "you wore a bowtie at your wedding, Grandpa." This may serve to prompt the relative to talk more about the picture/event.

16. The relative may talk inaccurately about the pictures. The child should not argue with him. Instead the child can suggest that they turn the page and look at the next picture. The child can also suggest that they read the sentences together. For instance, if the relative points at a picture of his wife and says, "That's my mother," the child can point to the sentence and say, "Look Grandpa, it says here, 'My wife's name is Mary Lou.' "

# Annotated Bibliography of Relevant Books for Children

Altman, L. J. (2002). *Singing with Momma Lou.* New York: Lee and Low Books, Inc.

*Summary:* Nine-year-old Tamika uses photographs, school yearbooks, movie ticket stubs, and other mementos to try to restore the memory of her grandmother, who has Alzheimer's disease. Ages 4–8.

Bahr, M. (1992). *The memory box.* Morton Grove, IL: Albert Whitman & Company.

*Summary:* When Gramps realizes he has Alzheimer's disease, he starts a memory box with his grandson, Zach, to keep memories of all the times they have shared. Ages 7–11.

Bauer, M. D. (1999). *An early winter.* New York: Clarion Books.

*Summary:* When 11-year-old Tim's beloved grandfather develops Alzheimer's disease, Tim tries to restore and save him by taking him out for a fishing adventure at the pond, but the outing turns into a disaster. Ages 9–12.

Fox, M. (1985). *Wilfrid Gordon McDonald Partridge.* Brooklyn, NY: Kane/Miller Book Publishers.

*Summary:* ("A Cranky Nell book.") A small boy tries to discover the meaning of "memory" so he can restore that of an elderly friend. Ages 4–8.

Frank, J. (1985). *Alzheimer's disease: The silent epidemic.* Minneapolis, MN: Lerner Publications Company.

*Summary:* This book introduces readers to AD by telling the story of Sarah, a typical victim, and the loving family that sees her through the long and fatal course of her illness. The book uses detailed diagrams to explain exactly what is happening to cause the symptoms of memory loss and confusion. Also, this book looks at the current medical research on the causes and possible cures for AD. Age 11+.

Frantti, A. (2002). *Grandma's cobwebs.* Clifton Park, NY: Dagney Publishing.

*Summary:* Claire's parents teach her facts about Alzheimer's disease. They don't, however, pay much attention to how Claire is feeling about the changes in her grandmother's behavior. Ages 4–8.

Graber, R. (1986). *Doc.* New York: Harper & Row Junior Books.

*Summary:* Over the course of an emotionally charged summer, a teenage boy from a large, unusual family learns to accept that his grandfather has Alzheimer's disease. Age 12+.

Guthrie, D. (1986). *Grandpa doesn't know it's me.* New York: Human Sciences Press, Inc.

*Summary:* This is a story, written from a child's point of view, of an experience with Alzheimer's disease. A little girl narrates the gradual changes in her grandfather and the family's recognition of and experiences with the disease. Ages 4–8.

Karkowsky, N. (1989). *Grandma's soup.* Toronto, Ontario: Kar-Ben Publishing.

*Summary:* Grandma suddenly starts to forget how to make chicken soup and her grandchildren's names. Ages 4–8.

Laminack, L. (1998). *The sunsets of Miss Olivia Wiggins.* Atlanta, GA: Peachtree Publishers.

*Summary:* This poignant tale of a woman residing in a nursing home, who seems to live more in a world of memories than in the present, gives voice to an often not-discussed element of aging. Ages 6–10.

Langston, L. (2004). *Remember, Grandma.* New York, NY: Viking Books.

*Summary:* A lyrical and simply drawn book of a granddaughter who watches her grandmother slowly forget things, but finds a way to help her remember and for the two to have a relationship. Ages 4–8.

McIntyre, C. (2005). *Flowers for Grandpa Dan: A gentle story to help children understand Alzheimer's disease.* St. Louis, MO: Thumbprint Press.

*Summary:* A poignant and perceptive account of a child coping with the loss of his beloved grandfather to Alzheimer's dementia. As Alzheimer's disease gradually changes Grandpa Dan, Grandson Danny learns there is one important thing that never changes. Ages 4–8.

Nelson, V. M. (1988). *Always Gramma.* New York: Putnam.

*Summary:* A loving grandchild describes what it is like when Gramma becomes increasingly confused and forgetful, to the point that she can no longer take care of herself. Ages 4–8.

Park, B. (2000). *The graduation of Jake Moon.* New York: Atheneum Books for Young Readers.

*Summary:* Fourteen-year-old Jake recalls how he has spent the last 4 years of his life watching his grandfather descend slowly but surely into the horrors of Alzheimer's disease. Ages 9–12.

Schwartz, N. (1998). *Old timers: The one that got away.* Downsview, Ontario: Tumbleweed Press.

*Summary:* After a visit with his grandfather who has Alzheimer's disease, a 10-year-old boy realizes how lucky he has been to know Pop and to share his stories. Ages 9–12.

Shecter, B. (1996). *Great-Uncle Alfred forgets.* New York: Harper Collins Publishers.

*Summary:* A young girl takes her great-uncle, who has Alzheimer's disease, for a walk and gently and patiently answers all his seemingly absurd questions. Ages 4–8.

Shriver, M. (2004). *What's happening to Grandpa?* New York: Little, Brown and Company.

*Summary:* This story takes a young girl through acceptance and a beginning understanding of her Grandpa's condition. Ages 4–8.

Swallow, P. C. (2003). *It only looks easy.* Brookfield, CT: Roaring Brook Press.

*Summary:* On the first day of seventh grade when Kat "borrows" a bicycle to go see her dog who was hit the day before by a woman with Alzheimer's disease, she learns about the serious consequences of impetuous actions and manages to make some new friends in the process. Ages 9–12.

Wild, M. (1995). *Remember me.* Morton Grove, IL: Albert Whitman & Company.

*Summary:* A warm and sensitive portrayal of memory loss and the joy that intergenerational relationships can bring, told from an elderly woman's point of view. Grandma is beginning to forget things or lose things, and her highly enthusiastic and loving granddaughter devises ways to help her remember with such devices as tying knots in her hanky and leaving notes everywhere. Ages 4–8.

Williams, C. L. (1998). *If I forget, you remember.* New York: Delacorte Press.

*Summary:* Twelve-year-old Elyse's plan to write an award-winning novel during the summer is interrupted when her grandmother, who has Alzheimer's disease, moves in with the family. Ages 9–12.

# References

Allen-Burge, R., Burgio, L., Bourgeois, M., Sims, R., & Nunnikhoven, J. (2001). Increasing communication among nursing home residents. *Journal of Clinical Geropsychology, 7*, 213–230.

Baddeley, A. (1992). Working memory. *Science, 255*, 556–559.

Baddeley, A. (1995). The psychology of memory. In A. D. Baddeley, B. A. Wilson, & F. N. Watts (Eds.), *Handbook of memory disorders (pp. 3–26)*. New York: Wiley.

Bourgeois, M. (1990). Enhancing conversation skills in Alzheimer's disease using a prosthetic memory aid. *Journal of Applied Behavior Analysis, 23*, 29–42.

Bourgeois, M. (1991, May). Improving the conversations of patients with Alzheimer's disease in nursing home settings. Paper presented at the Association for Behavior Analysis Conference, Atlanta, GA.

Bourgeois, M. (1992a). *Enhancing the conversations of memory-impaired persons: A memory aid workbook.* Gaylord, MI: Northern Speech Services, Inc.

Bourgeois, M. (1992b). Evaluating memory wallets in conversations with patients with dementia. *Journal of Speech and Hearing Research, 35*, 1344–1357.

Bourgeois, M. (1993). Effects of memory aids on the dyadic conversations of individuals with dementia. *Journal of Applied Behavior Analysis, 26*, 77–87.

Bourgeois, M. (1997). *My book of memories: A workbook to aid individuals with impairments of memory.* Gaylord, MI: Northern Speech Services, Inc.

Bourgeois, M. (2006). External aids. In D. K. Attix & K. Welsh-Bohmer (Eds.), *Geriatric neuropsychological assessment & intervention* (pp. 333–346). New York: Guilford Press.

Bourgeois, M., Burgio, L., Schulz, R., Beach, S., & Palmer, B. (1997). Modifying repetitive verbalization of community dwelling patients with AD. *The Gerontologist, 37*, 30–39.

Bourgeois, M., Camp, C., Rose, M., White, B., Malone, M., Carr, J., et al. (2003). A comparison of training strategies to enhance use of external aids by persons with dementia. *Journal of Communication Disorders, 36,* 361–379.

Bourgeois, M., Dijkstra, K., Burgio, L., & Allen, R. S. (2004). Communication skills training for nursing aides of residents with dementia: The impact of measuring performance. *Clinical Gerontologist, 27,* 119–138.

Bourgeois, M., Dijkstra, K., Burgio, L., & Allen-Burge, R. (2001). Memory aids as an AAC strategy for nursing home residents with dementia. *Augmentative and Alternative Communication, 17,* 196–210.

Bourgeois, M., Dijkstra, K., & Hickey, E. (2005). Impact of communicative interaction on measuring quality of life in dementia. *Journal of Medical Speech Language Pathology, 13,* 37–50.

Bourgeois, M., & Irvine, B. (1999). *Working with dementia: communication tools for professional caregivers.* CD-ROM and videotape in-service training programs available from ORCAS, Oregon Center for Applied Science, Inc., Eugene, OR.

Bourgeois, M., & Mason, L. A. (1996). Memory wallet intervention in an adult day care setting. *Behavioral Interventions: Theory and Practice in Residential and Community-Based Clinical Programs, 11,* 3–18.

Brush, J., & Camp, C. (1998a). Using spaced retrieval as an intervention during speech-language therapy. *Clinical Gerontologist, 19,* 51–64.

Brush, J., & Camp, C. (1998b). *A therapy technique for improving memory: Spaced retrieval.* Beachwood, OH: Menorah Park Center for Aging.

Buettner, L. (1999). Simple Pleasures: A multilevel sensorimotor intervention for nursing home residents with dementia. *American Journal of Alzheimer's Disease, Jan/Feb,* 41–52.

Buettner, L., & Martin, S. (1995). *Therapeutic recreation in the nursing home.* State College, PA: Venture Publishing.

Burdick, L. (2005). *The sunshine on my face.* Baltimore, MD: Health Professions Press.

Burgio, L., Allen-Burge, R., Roth, D., Bourgeois, M., Dijkstra, K., Gerstle, J., et al. (2001). Come talk with me: Improving communication between nursing assistants and nursing home residents during care routines. *The Gerontologist, 41,* 449–460.

Camp, C. J. (1999). *Montessori-based activities for persons with dementia. Vol 1.* Beachwood, OH: Menorah Park Center for the Aging.

Camp, C. J. (2005). Spaced retrieval: A case study in dissemination of a cognitive intervention for persons with dementia. In D. K. Attix & K. A. Welsch-Bohmner (Eds.), *Geriatric neuropsychological assessment and intervention.* New York: Guilford Press.

Camp, C., Bird, M., & Cherry, K. (2000). Retrieval strategies as a rehabilitation aid for cognitive loss in pathological aging. In R. D. Hill, L. Bäckman, & A. Neely (Eds.), *Cognitive rehabilitation in old age* (pp. 224–248). New York: Oxford University Press.

Dijkstra, K., & Bourgeois, M. (2004, July). Using life experiences in dementia: The teacher role. Paper presented at the Ninth International Conference on Language and Social Psychology, State College, PA.

Dijkstra, K., Bourgeois, M., Burgio, L., & Allen, R. (2002). Effects of communication training on the discourse of nursing home residents with dementia and their nursing assistants. *Journal of Medical Speech-Language Pathology, 10,* 143–157.

Dijkstra, K., Bourgeois, M., Petrie, G., Burgio, L., & Allen-Burge, R. (2002). My recaller is on vacation: Discourse analysis of nursing home residents with cognitive impairments. *Discourse Processes, 33,* 53–76.

Eisner, E. (2001). *Can Do activities for adults with Alzheimer's disease: Strength-based communication and programming.* Austin, TX: Pro-Ed.

Fogler, J., & Stern, L. (1988). *Improving your memory.* Baltimore, MD.: Johns Hopkins University Press.

Folstein, M. F., Folstein, S. E., & McHugh, P. R. (1975). "Minimental State": A practical method for grading the mental state of patients for the clinician. *Journal of Psychiatric Research, 12,* 189–198.

Hoerster, L., Hickey, E., & Bourgeois, M. (2001). Effects of memory aids on conversations between nursing home residents with dementia and nursing assistants. *Neuropsychological Rehabilitation, 11,* 399–427.

Hultsch, D., Hertzog, C., Small, B., & Dixon, R. (1999). Use it or lose it: Engaged lifestyle as a buffer of cognitive decline in aging. *Psychology & Aging, 14,* 245–263.

Irvine, A. B., Bourgeois, M., & Ary, D. V. (2003). An interactive multi-media program to train professional caregivers. *Journal of Applied Gerontology, 22,* 269–288.

Kapur, N. (1995). Memory aids in the rehabilitation of memory disordered patients. In A. D. Baddeley, B. A. Wilson, & F. N. Watts FN (Eds.), *Handbook of memory disorders (pp. 534–556).* Chichester, England: Wiley.

Lynch, B. (2002). Historical review of computer-assisted cognitive retraining. *Journal of Head Trauma Rehabilitation, 17,* 446–457.

Malone, M., Camp, C., & Rose, M. (2003, November). *The spaced-retrieval technique: A "Train the Trainer" program for rehabilitation staff.* Poster presented at the Gerontological Society of America annual conference, San Diego, CA.

Mackinnon, A., Christensen, H., Hofer, S., Korten, A., & Jorm, A. (2003). Use it and still lose it? The association between activity and cognitive performance established using latent growth techniques in a community sample. *Aging, Neuropsychology, & Cognition, 10,* 215–229.

Sohlberg, M. M., & Mateer, C. (2001). *Cognitive rehabilitation: An integrative neuropsychological approach.* New York: Guilford Press.

Sudol, E. (1999). *Look 'n cook microwave: Easy-to-make illustrated recipes.* Verona, WI: Attainment Company, Inc.

# Making Wearable Devices for Memory Aids

## *An Instructional Manual*

**Michelle S. Bourgeois, Ph.D., CCC-SLP**, Florida State University

*With* Ellen M. Hickey, Ph.D., CCC-SLP, Dalhousie University, and
Katinka Dijkstra, Ph.D., Florida State University
*Illustrations by* Christopher P. Reilly, Seattle, WA

## CONTENTS

## Introduction

The purpose of this manual is to provide families and other caregivers with ways to create devices that make memory aids more accessible for individuals with memory impairment. Individuals who have memory impairment are frequently supplied with a memory aid by a speech-language pathologist or other health care professional. Memory aids promote increased independence and improved quality of life. However, for this to be possible, the memory aids must be accessible to the individuals who need them. This manual provides caregivers with ways of making memory aids "wearable." This can be accomplished by making the memory aid small, lightweight, and portable and using an adaptive device to carry the memory aid.

Another issue regarding accessibility of memory aids in nursing homes is staff compliance with supplying the aids. Wearable memory aids should be included in individualized care plans, just as adaptive devices such as walkers, splints, eyeglasses, and hearing aids are. This would increase the awareness and compliance of staff members in making the prescribed memory aids available to their residents.

This manual provides ideas for devices, along with step-by-step instructions and pictures for making wearable memory aid devices. Included are vest pockets, wheelchair and walker bags, a necklace, and a belt. Feel free to adapt the ideas to your family member's or resident's needs. The only limit on making these devices is your own creativity!

# Vest Pocket

The vest pocket is a popular form of adaptive device for memory aids because it is easy to wear and easy to access the memory aid. For men, a suit vest can be used and worn over any kind of shirt or sweater. For women, a favorite vest can be used and worn over a dress or any kind of top. A clear plastic pocket is sewn onto the vest to carry the memory aid. The size of the pocket can be adjusted to match the shape and size of the vest. Just make sure the pocket is large enough to hold the memory aid. If your family member does not already own a vest that can be adapted, then one can be purchased at a thrift store (for example, Good Will or Salvation Army stores). Alternatively, fabric stores and craft shops often carry patterns or fabric printed with vest designs to

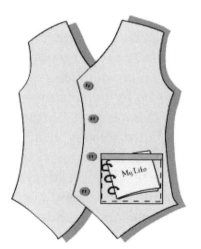

cut out and sew. These stores also sell the clear plastic by the yard.

## Materials Needed for Men's or Women's Vest

Craft plastic, $10'' \times 8''$

$10''$ double-fold bias binding tape in a color that matches the vest

Thread that matches the vest and bias tape

Scissors

Sewing machine

## Instructions

1. Place plastic on top of vest. Draw the shape of the lower part of the vest onto the plastic. Cut out the pocket shape $\frac{1}{4}''$ larger than the desired pocket on the sides and bottom edges.

2. Sew the double-fold bias binding tape to the top edge of the plastic.

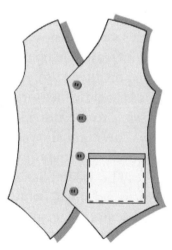

3. Fold $\frac{1}{4}''$ of the sides and bottom edge of the plastic to the wrong side. Press the $\frac{1}{4}''$ fold.

4. Edge stitch through the folded plastic onto the vest.

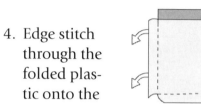

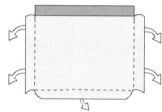

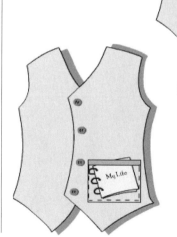

5. Put the memory book in the pocket and share it with your family member.

# Wheelchair and Walker Bags

Wheelchair bags are useful for those individuals who are nonambulatory. The bag can be attached to the wheelchair arm with Velcro straps to make it easily accessible for your family member or resident and for caregivers. Bags can also be made to fit on a variety of walkers for those individuals who are ambulatory with a walker.

## Wheelchair Bags

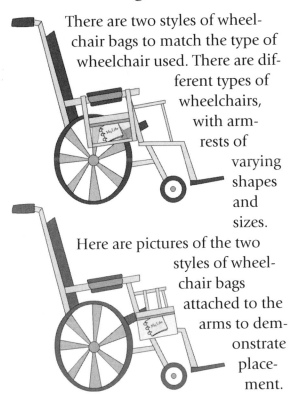

There are two styles of wheelchair bags to match the type of wheelchair used. There are different types of wheelchairs, with armrests of varying shapes and sizes.

Here are pictures of the two styles of wheelchair bags attached to the arms to demonstrate placement.

The exact proportions for the bag will depend on the shape and size of the wheelchair. The suggested dimensions on the following pages are for a bag to fit an average size wheelchair. You will need to measure the armrest of your family member's chair to determine exact proportions for the bag.

## Walker Bag

Walker bags are useful for those individuals who are ambulatory with a walker. The bag can be attached to the front bar of the walker with Velcro straps. This keeps the memory aid in view of your family member or resident and accessible to the caregivers. It is suggested that you follow the directions for wheelchair bag #1 (see next page) for use on a walker, although wheelchair bag #2 will also work.

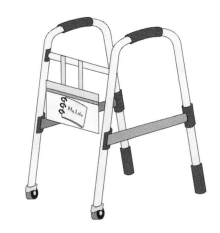

# Wheelchair/Walker Bag #1

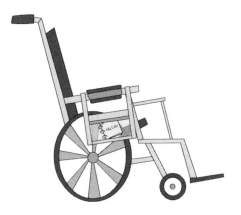

## Materials Needed for a 6″ × 10″ Bag

Cotton or cotton-blend fabric, 16″ × 16″

2 strips of Velcro, ¾″ × 3″

Craft plastic, 8″ × 5″

10″ double-fold bias binding tape in a color that matches the fabric

Thread that matches the bias tape and fabric

Scissors

Sewing machine

| | | Scrap 4″ x 10″ | Strap 3″ x 16″ | Strap 3″ x 16″ |
|---|---|---|---|---|
| 4″ | | | | |
| 6″ | | 6″ x 10″ | | |
| | | (fold) | | |
| 6″ | | 6″ x 10″ | | |
| | 10″ | | 3″ | 3″ |

## Instructions

1. Cut fabric as shown in the diagram

2. Or measure the length of the arm rest in front of the wheel and cut fabric 2″ longer than the desired length of the pocket, and 12″ wide. (Save the left-over fabric for the straps)

3. Cut plastic 5″ wide and 8″ long, or 1″ shorter than the desired length of the bag.

4. On the top and bottom of the fabric, fold ¼″ to the wrong side. Press folded edges.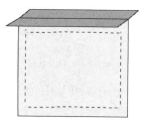

5. Fold the bias binding tape over the top edge of the plastic. Sew the double-fold bias binding tape to the top edge of the plastic.

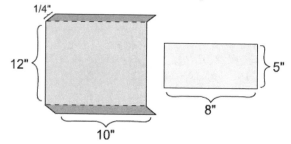

6. Fold the fabric in half, right sides together. Place plastic (bias tape edge down) between the 2 edges of fabric.

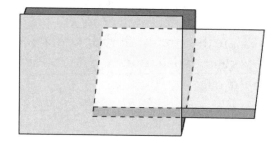

7. Sew together the fabric and the plastic along the edge (do not sew sides).

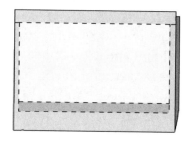

8. Turn fabric right-side out, with plastic on top of the fabric, and with the bottom (sewn) edge of the fabric turned up ½″.

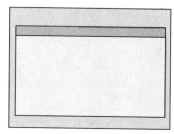

9. Cut the straps as shown in the diagram (16″ × 3″) or cut the leftover fabric to make straps. Press ¼″ of all edges to the wrong side.

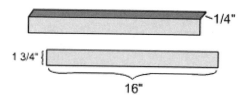

10. Fold the straps over the sides of the pocket, aligning the end of the strap with the bottom of the pocket, and overlapping the plastic at least ¼″.

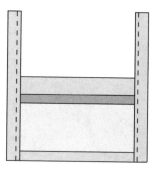

11. Sew the edges of the straps, starting at the top and sewing down the edges and onto the plastic pocket.

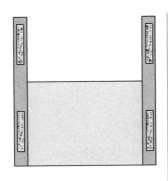

12. Sew one side of the Velcro pieces against the top part of the straps. Sew the other side of the Velcro pieces on the back side of the straps, aligned with the top edge of the bag.

13. Hang the bag from the wheelchair and insert the memory aid.

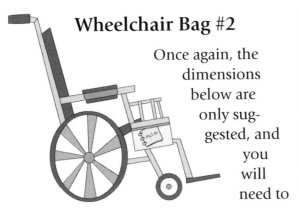

## Wheelchair Bag #2

Once again, the dimensions below are only suggested, and you will need to measure the wheelchair to determine exact dimensions for your family member's bag.

## Materials Needed for a 6″ × 8″ Bag

Cotton or cotton-blend fabric, 8″ × 17″

Craft plastic, 8″ × 5″

2 strips of Velcro, ¾″ × 3″

10″ double-fold bias binding tape

Thread that matches the bias tape and bag

Scissors

Sewing machine

| 2.5″ | 2.5″ | 6″ | 6″ | | 5″ |
|---|---|---|---|---|---|
| 8″ | | fabric | | 8″ | plastic 8″ |

## Instructions

1. Cut the fabric into 2 pieces that are 8″ × 6″ for the body of the bag, and 2 pieces that are 8″ × 2½″ for the straps. Fold ¼″ to the wrong side on the long edges of the straps, and the top edges of the body of the bag. Press all folded edges.

2. Fold the bias binding tape over the top edge of the plastic. Sew the bias binding tape to the top edge of the plastic.

3. Align the two pieces of fabric for the body of the bag, with right sides together. Insert the plastic between the fabric and align with the edges of the fabric. Sew the sides and bottom, leave the top edge open.

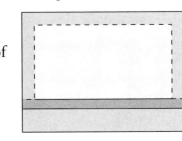

4. Turn the fabric right-side out, with the plastic pocket sitting on top, and the sewn edge forming the bottom of the bag.

5. Fold the 2 strap pieces in half lengthwise. Sew the edges of the straps.

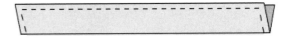

6. Insert 1″ of the end of each strap between the 2 pieces of fabric at the top of the bag. Sew the top edge of the bag.

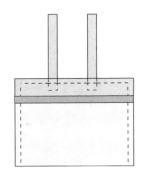

7. Sew the Velcro pieces to the top of the strap and back of the bag.

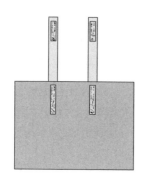

8. Hang the bag on the chair and insert the memory book in the pocket.

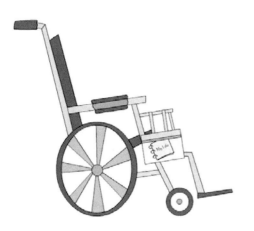

## Waist Pack

The waist pack is a convenient bag for those who are ambulatory without a walker. This bag will allow your family member to keep the memory aid easily accessible without interfering with mobility. A commercially available waist pack could also be used, but the disadvantage is that the pocket will not be clear, and

your family member or the caregivers may forget that it contains the memory aid. This bag is similar to wheelchair bag #2, but with some modifications for the strap.

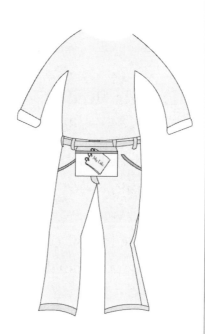

## Materials Needed for a 6″ × 8″ Bag

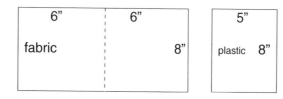

Cotton or cotton-blend fabric, 12″ × 8″, and a strip 3″ wide by 2″ longer than your family member's waist dimension

Craft plastic, 8″ × 5″

1 strip of Velcro, 1″ × 3″

8″ double-fold bias binding tape

Thread that matches the bias tape and bag

Scissors

Sewing machine

## Instructions

1. Cut the fabric into 2 pieces that are 8″ × 6″ for the body of the bag, and 1 strap piece that is 2″ longer than your family member's waist dimension by 3″ wide. Fold ¼″ to the wrong side on the long edge of the strap, and the top edges of the body of the bag. Press all folded edges.

2. Fold the bias tape over the top edge of the plastic. Sew the bias tape to the top edge of the plastic.

3. Align the two pieces of fabric for the body of the bag, with right sides together. Insert the plastic between

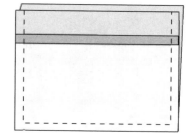

the fabric and align with the edges of the fabric. Sew the bottom and side edges of the fabric and plastic, leaving the top open.

4. Turn the fabric right-side out, with the plastic pocket sitting on top, and the sewn edge forming the bottom of the bag.

5. Fold the strap length-wise over the top of the bag so the bag is centered in the middle.

6. Sew the edges of the strap, going through the top of the bag.

7. Sew the Velcro to the ends of the strap— one on the front and one on the back side of the strap, so that when the strap is wrapped around the waist, the pieces will come together.

8. Put the memory book in the bag and put it on your family member.

## Apron

Aprons can be adapted for men or women. Any style of apron will work fine. It is easiest to use an apron that your family member owns, or you can buy one (*note*: most thrift stores have a wide variety of aprons). In either case, you can simply sew a pocket onto the apron. Alternatively, you can sew an apron, using a commercially available pattern, and adding a clear pocket to it. Below are instructions for sewing a pocket onto an apron.

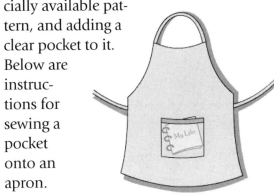

## Materials Needed for Apron

8″ × 6″ piece of craft plastic

8″ strip double-fold bias binding tape in a color that matches the apron

Scissors

Sewing machine (or needle and thread)

Thread in a color that matches the apron and bias tape

## Instructions

1. Fold the bias tape over the top edge of the plastic. Stitch the bias tape to the top edge of the plastic.

2. Press ¼″ to the wrong side on the bottom and sides of the plastic.

3. Position the plastic on the apron. Stitch the bottom and side edges of the plastic to the apron.

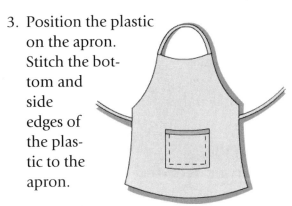

4. Put the apron on your family member and insert the memory book.

## Belt

Belts can be adapted or crafted for both men and women. The memory aid can be attached to a favorite belt by hanging the aid from a coiled cord or bias binder strap. Make sure to have the cord or straps long enough so that your family member can comfortably use the memory aid while still attached to the belt. If your family member does not have a belt available, then you can make a fabric belt following the instructions below. You will need to measure your family member's waist to determine exact measurements for the materials listed.

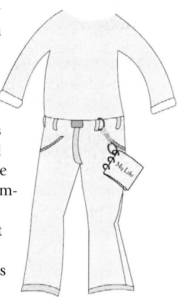

## Materials Needed for a Belt

5" wide cotton or cotton-blend fabric, with length 4" longer than your family member's waist

Elastic, length equal to your family member's waist

1 strip of Velcro 1" × 3"

Scissors

Sewing machine (or needle and thread)

Thread that matches fabric

Plastic spiral cord (like a key chain)

## Instructions

1. Use a belt or measuring tape to determine the desired length of the fabric belt.

2. Cut the elastic equal to your family member's waist dimension. Cut the fabric 4" longer than your family member's waist dimension.

3. Fold the fabric in half lengthwise, with the right sides together. Stitch the edges of the fabric.

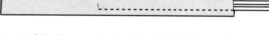

4. Turn the fabric right-side out. Place the elastic inside the fabric.

5. Fold the ends inside ¼". Stitch the ends.

6. Sew one side of Velcro to each end of the belt, one on the top and the other on the bottom of the belt.

7. Attach the plastic spiral cord to the belt. Attach one ring of the memory aid to the spiral cord. Put the belt on your family member.

## Necklace

The necklace is a simple alternative for women. Any long, sturdy chain or beaded necklace that your family member owns can be used, or you can buy or make one. You could also purchase a plastic cord used in many workplaces for wearing photo identification. The necklace can be made from fabric or ribbon. If making a fabric necklace, follow the instructions to make the belt, but do not use elastic, and make it half as wide. Instructions are provided for making the ribbon necklace.

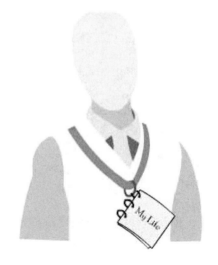

## Materials Needed for Necklace

Lightweight fabric or ribbon, suggested size approximately 26″ × ¾″ (or so the memory aid rests approximately 4″ above the navel)

1″ × ½″ Velcro strip

Decorative beads

Thread that matches ribbon

## Instructions

1. Cut ribbon to desired length.

2. String decorative beads (optional).

3. Sew Velcro to the ends of the ribbon, one piece on the top and the other piece on the bottom edge.

4. Loop the binder ring of the memory aid through the ribbon.

5. Share the memory aid and necklace with your family member.

## Other Attachments

You may think of other ways to add pockets to clothing, or to use attachments to keep memory aids with your family member. One more adaptive device is the use of a spiral cord key chain to attach the memory aid to a wheelchair, walker, or belt loop. Below are some pictures of the use of spiral cords. Feel free to use your knowledge of your family member's tastes to be creative and devise your own adaptive devices. Once again, the only limit is your own imagination!

**Spiral cord on wheelchair**

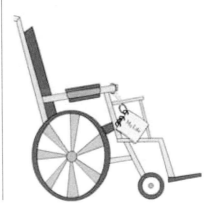

### Spiral cord on walker

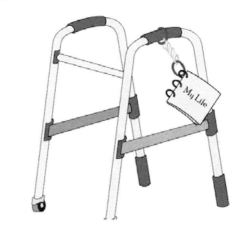

### Spiral cord on belt loop

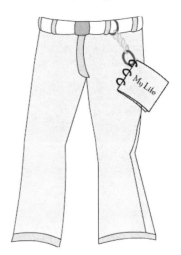

This project was supported by a grant from the National Institute on Aging (R01AG13008) to Florida State University.

# Additional Memory Aid Tools

## CONTENTS

# Making Memory Aids
*Family Caregiver Instructions*

1. Complete a **Memory Aid Information Form.**
2. Make a written list of all possible sentences to include in the memory aid.
3. Chose an appropriate number of written sentences or reproducible pages to include in the memory aid for your family member.
4. Find family pictures that clearly illustrate each of the sentences. Magazine pictures and other souvenirs or familiar items, such as maps, concert programs, ticket stubs, invitations, greeting cards, etc., can also be included to illustrate the pages.
5. Choose the size of memory aid that you feel is most appropriate for your family member. Memory Wallets are recommended for persons who live at home and still go on outings outside of the home; Memory Books are better for persons who are housebound or in nursing homes, and who may have trouble turning small pages. Wearable memory wallets are also valuable in the nursing home or assisted living setting.
6. Assemble supplies needed to make memory aid. Remember the scissors, glue, and a black ink pen.
7. Print sentences in black ink and large letters, or use your computer to type the words on the pages.
8. Trim and paste pictures onto relevant pages.
9. Slip book pages into clear plastic page protectors or laminate wallet pages. Using a hole-punch, make holes for each wallet page.
10. Put all book pages in 3-ring notebook and wallet pages into wallet with 1 or more rings.
11. Read the **Guidelines for Having a Satisfying Conversation.**
12. Share the memory aid with its new owner.

# Guidelines for Having a Satisfying Conversation

1. *Ask* the person to have a conversation with you.

   "Mary, I'd really like to talk with you today. Would you mind if I sat down beside you?"

2. *Guide* the conversation onto specific topics and *redirect* the conversation back to the topic when the person begins to ramble.

   "Mary, let's talk about your family now, please tell me all about them."

3. *Reassure* the person and *help out* when he or she gets stuck or can't find a word.

   "That's ok, Bob; what else can you tell me about your life?"

4. *Smile* and *act interested* in whatever the person is talking about even if you're not quite sure what is being said.

5. *Thank* the person for talking with you.

## What to AVOID during conversations

- *DO NOT quiz* the person or ask lots of specific questions

   "Now who is this person? I know you know who she is!"

- *DO NOT correct* or *contradict* something that was stated as a fact even if you know it's wrong.

   "No, that's not John. That's Jason, remember, your grandson Jason?"

# Reminder Cards

*Using Written Cues in the Home and Nursing Home*

When a question is repeated a few seconds after you have just answered it, a **Reminder Card** may help to keep the information in mind. Follow these easy steps for successful remembering:

1. State the answer to the question or concern.

2. Write the answer on an index card or notepad.

3. Read the card aloud with the person and give it to him or her.

4. When the question is repeated, DO NOT say the answer, INSTEAD say, "Read the card."

5. Do this each time the question is repeated.

## Examples

Q. When am I going to the store?
A. **I am going to the store after lunch** (write this on the card).

Q. Where are we going?
A. **We are going to church** (write this on the card).

Q. Where is my paycheck?
A. **My money is safe in the bank** (write this on the card).

## Helpful Hints

- **Print a clear message.**
  Use large print. Use a few, simple, positive words.
- **Make the message personal.**
  Use personal pronouns (I, my, we) in the message.
- **Read the message aloud.**
  If there are reading errors, change the message.

# Reproducible Memory Booklet for Children to Make

The following pages can be copied, then folded in half, and stapled in the middle to make a booklet. Additional pages can be included for children to illustrate with drawings and other pictures. Encourage the child to decorate the cover and personalize the Memory Booklet for the relative or friend with memory impairment.

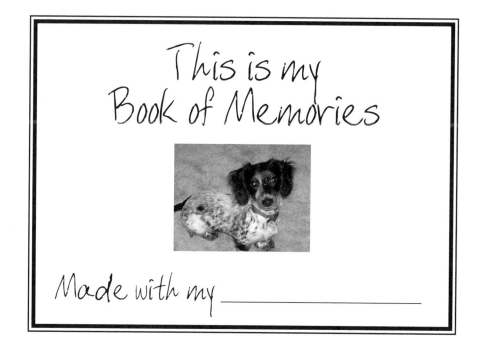

This is my
Book of Memories

Made with my _____

My name is_____

_____

I was born _____

_____

I love _____

_____

My favorite _____

is _____

# My children are _____

_____

# My grandchildren are_____

_____

I love _____

_____

My favorite _____

is_____

# This is my Book of Memories

Made with

_____

# Information and Assessment Forms

## CONTENTS

# Memory Aid Information Form

*Please complete this biographical information for:*

Name _____

Nickname _____

## Family Information

### MOTHER

Name _____

Date of Birth _____

Birthplace _____

Date of Death _____

### FATHER

Name _____

Date of Birth _____

Birthplace _____

Date of Death _____

**BROTHERS** (*names*) _____

_____

_____

**SISTERS** (*names*) _____

_____

_____

### WIFE/HUSBAND

Name _____

Date of Birth _____

Birthplace _____

Date of Marriage _____

Location of Marriage (city, state) _____

Date of Death (if applicable) _____

**CHILDREN** (*names*)

1 _____  3 _____

2 _____  4 _____

**SPOUSE OF CHILDREN** (*include married name for daughters*)

1 _____  3 _____

2 _____  4 _____

**GRANDCHILDREN**

1 _____  6 _____

2 _____  7 _____

3 _____  8 _____

4 _____  9 _____

5 _____  10 _____

What are the current occupations of these children:

1 _____  3 _____

2 _____  4 _____

Where are the children and grandchildren currently living (city, state)?

1 _____  3 _____

2 _____  4 _____

## Your Family Member's Life History

Date of Birth _____ Place of Birth _____

Childhood home (city, state) _____

High School _____ College _____

**MILITARY SERVICE**

Branch _____ When _____

**OCCUPATION(S)** WHEN

_____ _____

_____ _____

**SPECIAL HONORS/AWARDS**

_____

**HOBBIES, FAVORITE LEISURE ACTIVITIES** *(past and/or present)*

_____

**PLACES LIVED AS AN ADULT**                When

_____

**CLUBS, SOCIAL ORGANIZATIONS**             Held office?

_____

**CHURCH OR TEMPLE**

_____

**CHURCH OR TEMPLE RELATED ACTIVITIES OR INVOLVEMENTS** *(for example, deacon, choir, etc.)*

_____

_____

**FAVORITE PETS** *(past and/or present)*

_____

**MEMORABLE VACATIONS**

Where _____

When _____

With whom _____

**BEST FRIENDS**

_____

**ANY OTHER MEMORABLE EVENTS, DETAILS**

_____

**CHALLENGING BEHAVIORS** (*Describe any other specific problems you are having and how often they occur.*
*Example: My mother asks to go to church every 10 minutes.*)

_____

_____

_____

_____

**DAILY SCHEDULE** (*Please complete a daily schedule for your family member including all routine activities*)

| Usual Daily Schedule | Special Activities |
|---|---|
| 7:00 a.m. _____ | _____ |
| 7:30 a.m. _____ | _____ |
| 8:00 _____ | _____ |
| 8:30 _____ | _____ |
| 9:00 _____ | _____ |
| 9:30 _____ | _____ |
| 10:00 _____ | _____ |
| 10:30 _____ | _____ |
| 11:00 _____ | _____ |
| 11:30 _____ | _____ |
| 12 noon _____ | _____ |
| 12:30 p.m. _____ | _____ |
| 1:00 p.m. _____ | _____ |
| 1:30 _____ | _____ |

**DAILY SCHEDULE** (*Continued*)

2:00 _____

2:30 _____

3:00 _____

3:30 _____

4:00 _____

4:30 _____

5:00 _____

5:30 _____

6:00 _____

6:30 _____

7:00 _____

7:30 _____

8:00 _____

8:30 _____

9:00 _____

9:30 _____

10:00 _____

10:30 _____

11:00 _____

11:30 _____

12 midnight _____

Any other activities which your family member participates in during his/her spare time but which is not part of the daily schedule?

_____

_____

# Memory Aid Information Form for Nursing Homes

Resident Name _____ Room # _____

Roommate _____

Friends _____

Breakfast: time _____ favorite foods _____

Lunch: time _____ favorite foods _____

Dinner: time _____ favorite foods _____

Location of meals _____

**DAILY ACTIVITIES** (*what activity, with whom, location, who takes client to the activity and any other information pertaining to daily schedule*)

Approximate morning wake up time _____ Approximate bed time _____

Every day _____
_____

Monday _____

Tuesday _____

Wednesday _____

Thursday _____

Friday _____

Saturday _____

Sunday _____

Family who visit _____

Other family _____

**STAFF MEMBERS** (*name and activity*)

_____

_____

_____

Other Information: _____

_____

**Likes**

_____

_____

**Dislikes**

_____

_____

**INTERESTS AND HOBBIES**

_____

_____

_____

# Orientation Assessment Form

## ASSESSING THE ORIENTATION BEHAVIORS OF

*(name)*

| PAST BEHAVIORS *(for location/profession)* | | DESIRED BEHAVIORS *(for location/activities)* | |
|---|---|---|---|
| **Person:** | Supports: | **Person:** | Supports: |
| **Place:** | | **Place:** | |
| **Time:** | | **Time:** | |

# Personal Wants, Needs, and Safety Assessment Form

## ASSESSING THE WANTS, NEEDS, SAFETY OF

*(name)*

**ENVIRONMENT:**    Home    Hospital    Assisted Living    Nursing Home    *(circle one)*

**WANTS** *(The expression of personal preferences, likes and dislikes)*

| Likes | Dislikes |
|-------|----------|
|       |          |

**NEEDS** *(The satisfaction of physical comforts and emotional needs)*

| Physical | Emotional |
|----------|-----------|
| Pain     |           |

**SAFETY** *(The prevention of harm to oneself or others)*

Medication

Falls prevention

Eating

Personal hygiene

**ENVIRONMENTAL CONSTRAINTS**

**EMERGENCY CONTACTS**

# Graphic Art and Supply Sources

## Pictures and Clip-Art

**Microsoft** (2006). Microsoft Office Online.

**Attainment Company, Inc.,** P.O. Box 930160, Verona, WI 53593-0160
    Phone: 800-327-4269, Fax: 800-942-3865
    e-mail: info@attainmentcompany.com; Website: www.attainmentcompany.com
    Products:  Life in Focus CD (Royalty-free photos in context)
              Personal Success CD, Community Success CD
              Picture Cue Dictionary
              Shopping List Generator CD
              Picture Prompt Cards and Stickers
              Picture-Based Scheduling
              Many more . . .

**Mayer-Johnson LLC,** P.O. Box 1579, Solana Beach, CA 92075-7579
    Toll free: 800-588-4548
    Phone: 858-550-0084, Fax: 858-550-0449
    E-mail: mayerj@mayer-johnson.com; Website: www.mayer-johnson.com
    Products:  Boardmaker Symbols
              (over 3,000 symbols in bitmap format)
              Boardmaker Photo/Symbol Bundle
              (4,000 picture symbols, 2,200 sign language
              symbols, and 2,700 photographs)

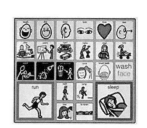

**Crestwood Communication Aids, Inc.,** P.O. Box 090107, Milwaukee, WI 53209-0107
   Phone: 414-352-5678, Fax: 414-352-5679
   E-mail: crestcomm@aol.com; Website: www.communicationaids.com
   Products: Picture Card Kits
            Casual Dining Passport®
            Supermarket Shopping Passport®
            Talking Pictures®
            Community Living Needs

**Health Passport®**

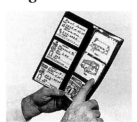
headache

**Large Porta Book**

**Interactive Therapeutics, Inc.,** P.O. Box 1805, Stow, OH 44224-0805
   Toll free: 800-253-5111(USA only), Phone: 330-923-7500, Fax: 330-923-3030
   E-mail: info@interactivetherapy.com; Website: www.interactivetherapy.com
   Products: Picture Communicators
            Daily Communicator
            My Medicines Wallet Card
            My Appointments Wallet Card
            Critical Communicator
            Table Chat Card Sets

**Daily Communicator®**

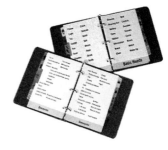

**Picture Communicators®**

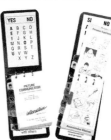

## Other Memory Book Supplies

**Office supply stores:** Photo albums, 3-ring binders, plastic page protectors
            Talking photo albums
            Talking photo album with recorder; manufacturers: CompUSA, Sears,
               Augmentative Communication, Inc. (www.augcominc.com),
               Brookstone (www.brookstone.com).

# ORDER FORM
# MEMORY BOOKS AND OTHER GRAPHIC CUING SYSTEMS

**My Order:**    Please send me ____ copies of **Memory Books and Other Graphic Cuing Systems**

at $32.95 each, plus $5.00 shipping and handling*

Total Payment:  $_____

\* Shipping and handling for 2 or more books is 10% of product total.

Shipping rates are for UPS Ground delivery within the continental U.S.

## SHIPPING INFORMATION

Name _____

Title _____

Organization _____

Street Address _____
(UPS cannot ship to P.O. boxes)

City/State/ZIP _____

Daytime phone (____)_____

Shipping address (check one):  ❑ Residential    ❑ Commercial

Email address _____
❑ I'd like to receive email updates about special offers or new products. My email will not be shared with another party.

Tell us more about your work setting (check one):

❑ Residential care      ❑ Community college/voc school      ❑ Acute clinical/medical
❑ Library               ❑ 4-Year college/grad school        ❑ Community
❑ Association/           ❑ Distance Learning
  foundation

## METHOD OF PAYMENT

❑ Check enclosed (payable to Health Professions Press)
❑ Purchase order attached (add 2% to product total for handling fee)
❑ Credit card:  ____ MasterCard  ____ VISA  ____ American Express

Card no. _____  Exp. date _____

Signature _____

**Return Form to:**
**Health Professions Press**
**P.O. Box 10624**
**Baltimore, MD  21285-0624**
**Toll-Free: 888-337-8808**
**FAX: 410-337-8539 • Phone: 410-337-9585**
**www.healthpropress.com**

**CONTACT US FOR INFORMATION ON QUANTITY DISCOUNTS**

Price may be higher outside the U.S and may be subject to change without notice.

**LIST CODE: ZMB**